Soft Tissue Sarcomas: New Developments in the Multidisciplinary Approach to Treatment

Cancer Treatment and Research

WILLIAM L. MCGUIRE, *series editor*

Soft Tissue Sarcomas: New Developments in the Multidisciplinary Approach to Treatment

edited by

Herbert M. Pinedo
Department of Medical Oncology
Free University Hospital
Amsterdam, The Netherlands

Jaap Verweij
Department of Medical Oncology
Rotterdam Cancer Institute
Rotterdam, The Netherlands

Herman D. Suit
Department of Radiation Medicine
Massachusetts General Hospital
Harvard Medical School
Boston, Massachusetts, U.S.A.

1991 **KLUWER ACADEMIC PUBLISHERS**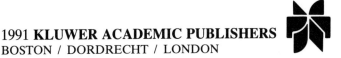
BOSTON / DORDRECHT / LONDON

Distributors for North America:
Kluwer Academic Publishers
101 Philip Drive
Assinippi Park
Norwell, Massachusetts 02061 U.S.A.

Distributors for all other countries:
Kluwer Academic Publishers Group
Distribution Centre
Post Office Box 322
3300 AH Dordrecht, THE NETHERLANDS

Library of Congress Cataloging-in-Publication Data

Soft tissue sarcomas: new developments in the multidisciplinary approach to
    treatment/edited by Herbert M. Pinedo, Jaap Verweij, and Herman D.
    Suit.
        p.   cm.—(Cancer treatment and research; 56)
    Includes bibliographical references and index.
    ISBN 0-7923-1139-6
    1. Sarcoma—Treatment.   I. Pinedo, H. M.   II. Verweij, J. (Jaap)
III. Suit, Herman D. (Herman Day), 1929–   .   IV. Series: Cancer
treatment and research; v. 56.
    [DNLM: 1. Sarcoma—therapy.   2. Soft Tissue Neoplasms—therapy.
W1 CA693 v. 56/   /WD 375 S681105]
RC280.C65S65   1991
616.99′4—dc20
DNLM/DLC
for Library of Congress   91–7002
                                                                                CIP

Cancer Treatment and Research is indexed in the National Library of
Medicine MEDLARS System.

PRINTED IN THE UNITED STATES OF AMERICA.

Contents

Cancer Treatment and Research

Foreword

Where do you begin to look for a recent, authoritative article on the diagnosis or management of a particular malignancy? The few general oncology textbooks are generally out of date. Single papers in specialized journals are informative, but seldom comprehensive; these are more often preliminary reports on a very limited number of patients. Certain general journals frequently publish good in-depth reviews of cancer topics, and published symposium lectures are often the best overviews available. Unfortunately, these reviews and supplements appear sporadically, and the reader can never be sure when a topic of special interest will be covered.

Cancer Treatment and Research is a series of authoritative volumes that aim to meet this need. It is an attempt to establish a critical mass of oncology literature covering virtually all oncology topics, which is revised frequently to keep the coverage up to date, and which is easily available on a single library shelf or by a single personal subscription.

We have approached the problem in the following fashion: first, by dividing the oncology literature into specific subdivisions, such as lung cancer, genitourinary cancer, pediatric oncology, etc.; and second, by asking eminent authorities in each of these areas to edit a volume on the specific topic on an annual or biannual basis. Each topic and tumor type is covered in a volume appearing frequently and predictably, discussing current diagnosis, staging, markers, all forms of treatment modalities, basic biology, and more.

In *Cancer Treatment and Research*, we have an outstanding group of editors, each having made a major commitment to bring to this new series the very best literature in his or her field. Kluwer Academic Publishers has made an equally major commitment to the rapid publication of high-quality books and to worldwide distribution.

Where can you go to quickly find a recent authoritative article on any major oncology problem? We hope that *Cancer Treatment and Research* provides an answer.

WILLIAM L. MCGUIRE
Series Editor

Preface

One of the major issues in the optimal treatment of soft tissue sarcomas is the necessity of treatment planning within the framework of a multidisciplinary approach. Fortunately, there is a tendency to having increasing numbers of patients discussed in multidisciplinary teams prior to the initial treatment. This fourth volume on soft tissue sarcomas in the series *Cancer Treatment and Research* reflects the multidisciplinary approach with a focus on recent developments.

The availability of new histopathology techniques has further increased the importance of the histopathologist in providing estimates of the prognosis of the patient as well as providing data for the planning of a treatment strategy. Further data for this strategy will be provided by diagnostic imaging. In this field, the role of magnetic resonance imaging has been further defined.

Of utmost importance is the recent trend towards concensus in staging. The modification of the AJC staging system brings the possibility of one single-staging system within reach in the next decade.

As surgery still provides the only chance for cure, the importance of being as sparing as possible is obvious. For this reason, radiotherapy has been applied with success. The introduction of relatively new radiation techniques is therefore observed with interest. Different schedules of combination of surgery with radiotherapy, sometimes also with chemotherapy, now have a high rate of efficacy in local control. Nevertheless, many patients will develop distant metastases.

The need for effective treatment of systemic disease is therefore even more obvious now than it was before. Unfortunately, systemic treatment is still bound to limitations. There are only a few truely active drugs, the most important being doxorubicin, ifosfamide, and DTIC. Whether standard-dose single-agent chemotherapy is as good as combination chemotherapy may be determined in the next few years.

The lack of efficacy of adjuvant chemotherapy with the drugs presently available has definitively been shown. However, chemotherapy may have an important role in the preoperative treatment of soft tissue sarcomas, although the optimal method of administration has yet to be defined, and the combination with other modalities, such as a.o. hyperthermia, may offer theoretical benefits.

Although the present volume focuses on new developments, previously obtained data are also briefly reviewed. With this in mind, we have invited a number of new authors to contribute to the present volume in order to extend the reader's scope in regard to the present state of the art. We would like to thank all the authors for their appreciated contribution.

H.M. Pinedo, H.D. Suit, and J. Verweij
Editors

Contributing Authors

BOTTI, C., Department of Surgical Oncology, Regina Elena Cancer Institute, Vie Regina Elena 291, Rome 00161, Italy

BRAMWELL, Vivien H.C., Department of Medical Oncology, London Regional Cancer Centre, 391 South Street, London, Ontario N6A 4G5, Canada

CARLINI, S., Department of Surgical Oncology, Regina Elena Cancer Institute, Vie Regina Elena 291, Rome 00161, Italy

CAVALIERE, F., Department of Surgical Oncology, Regina Elena Cancer Institute, Vie Regina Elena 291, Rome 00161, Italy

CAVALIERE, R., Department of Surgical Oncology, Regina Elena Cancer Institute, Vie Regina Elena 291, Rome 00161, Italy

COSTA, Jose, Institut Universitaire de Pathologie, Universite de Lausanne, Rue du Bugnon 25, CH-1011 Lausanne, Switzerland

DI FILIPPO, Franco, Department of Surgical Oncology, Regina Elena Cancer Institute, Vie Regina Elena 291, Rome 00161, Italy

GIANNARELLI, D., Department of Surgical Oncology, Regina Elena Cancer Institute, Vie Regina Elena 291, Rome 00161, Italy

GRAZIANO, F., Department of Surgical Oncology, Regina Elena Cancer Institute, Vie Regina Elena 291, Rome 00161, Italy

GEBHART, Mark C., Orthopedic Oncology Unit, Massachussetts General Hospital, Harvard Medical School, Boston, MA 02114, U.S.A.

GUILLOU, L., Institut Universitaire de Pathologie, Universite de Lausanne, Rue du Bugnon 25, CH-1011 Lausanne, Switzerland

HERRLIN, Kristian, Central Department of Diagnostic Radiology, University Hospital, S-22185 Lund, Sweden

KREMENTZ, Edward T., Department of Surgery, Tulane University School of Medicine, 1430 Tulane Avenue, New Orleans, LA 70112, U.S.A.

KUN, Larry E., Department of Radiotherapy, St. Jude Children's Research Hospital, 332 North Lauderdale, Memphis, TN 38101, U.S.A.

MANKIN, Henry J., Orthopedic Oncology Unit, Massachusetts General Hospital, Harvard Medical School, Boston, MA 02114, U.S.A.

MERTENS, Wilson C., Department of Medical Oncology, London Regional Cancer Centre, 391 South Street, London, Ontario N6A 4G5, Canada

MEYER, Michael, Department of Surgery, Tulane University School of Medicine, 1430 Tulane Avenue, New Orleans, LA 70112, U.S.A.

MUCHMORE, James H., Department of Surgery, Tulane University School of Medicine, 1430 Tulane Avenue, New Orleans, LA 70112, U.S.A.

PINEDO, Herbert M., Department of Medical Oncology, Free University Hospital and Netherlands Cancer Institute, De Boelelaan 1117, 1081 HV Amsterdam, The Netherlands

PETTERSON, Holger, Central Department of Diagnostic Radiology, University Hospital S-22185 Lund, Sweden

PRATT, Charles B., Department of Hematology/Oncology, St. Jude Children's Research Hospital, 332 North Lauderdale, Memphis, TN 38101, U.S.A.

RUSSELL, William O., 5601 N.E. 14th Avenue, Fort Lauderdale, FL 33334, U.S.A.

SUIT, Herman D., Department of Radiation Medicine, Massachussetts General Hospital Harvard Medical School, Boston, MA 02114, U.S.A.

SPRINGFIELD, Dempsey S., Orthopedic Oncology Unit, Massachussetts General Hospital, Harvard Medical School, Boston, 02114, U.S.A.

VERWEIJ, Jaap, Department of Medical Oncology, Rotterdam Cancer Institute, Groene Hilledijk 301, 3075 EA Rotterdam, The Netherlands

WEDDINGTON, William W., Department of Psychiatry, University of Illinois at Chicago, 912 South Wood Street, Chicago, IL 60612, U.S.A.

WILLET, Christopher G., Department of Radiation Medicine, Massachussetts General Hospital, Harvard Medical School, Boston, MA 02114, U.S.A.

List of Abbreviations

ACS	=	American College of Surgeons
ADIC	=	Doxorubicin/DTIC
AIDS	=	Acquired immune deficiency syndrome
AJC	=	American Joint Commission for Cancer Staging and End Results Reporting
b.w.	=	Body weight
CDDP	=	Cisplatin
CT	=	Computer tomography
CTX	=	Cyclophosphamide
CYVADIC	=	Cyclophosphamide/ vincristine/doxorubicin/DTIC
DACT	=	Actinomycin D
DDFS	=	Distant (metastases) disease free survival
DFS	=	Disease free survival
DM	=	Distant metastases
DSA	=	Digital subtraction angiography
DTIC	=	Dacarbazine
DX	=	Doxorubicin
ECOG	=	Eastern Cooperative Oncology Group
EORTC	=	European Organization on Treatment and Research of Cancer
FN	=	Fast neutrons
FNA	=	Fine needle aspiration
HAP	=	Hyperthermic antiblastic perfusion
IFOS	=	Ifosfamide
IGR	=	Institute Gustave Roussy
IL-2	=	Interleukin-2
IORT	=	Intraoperative radiation therapy
LC	=	Local control
LE	=	Lower extremity
L-PAM	=	Melphalan
MDAH	=	MD Anderson Hospital
MDR	=	Multidrug resistance phenotype
MFH	=	Malignant fibrous histiocytoma

MGH	=	Massachusetts General Hospital
MPNST	=	Malignant peripheral nerve sheath tumor
MMS	=	Mixed mesodermal sarcoma
MR	=	Magnetic resonance
MTS	=	Musculoskeletal Tumor Society
NCI	=	National Cancer Institute
OS	=	Overall survival
RFS	=	Relapse free survival
RPMI	=	Roswell Park Memorial Institute
SCC	=	Squamous cell cancer
SF 2	=	Survival fraction after 2 Gy
STS	=	Soft tissue sarcoma
SWOG	=	South West Oncology Group
TNF	=	Tumor necrosis factor
UCSF	=	University Center State of Florida
VCR	=	Vincristine
VRN	=	Von Recklinghausen's neurofibromatosis

Soft Tissue Sarcomas: New Developments in the Multidisciplinary Approach to Treatment

1. Pathology of Soft Tissue Sarcomas

Jose Costa and L. Guillou

The information derived from the pathological study of tissue is central to the management of patients presenting with soft tissue lesions. The histological diagnosis can be derived from good sections obtained from an excision or an incisional biopsy. A clinical history and knowledge of the radiological and clinical findings are helpful and sometimes essential. A fine needle aspiration (FNA) is an efficient way to orient the diagnosis (e.g., lymphoma vs. mesenchymal lesion) and a good approach to the planning of diagnostic surgery. FNA is also a good technique to establish the diagnosis of recurrent disease. However, accurate histological typing and grading of most lesions require a detailed and generous sampling of the entire lesion. Whenever possible, tissue should be put aside for electron microscopy and immunohistochemistry on frozen sections.

Because of the diverse histological appearances of lesions occuring in the soft tissues, histological diagnosis and classification can be challenging. In the hands of competent pathologists and with the use of ancillary techniques, at least 90% of tumors and tumor-like lesions can be accurately diagnosed and classified.

The most difficult area for the diagnostician remains that of "borderline lesions" (Table 1). Borderline can refer to two types of lesions: one is benign, but mimics malignancy (pseudosarcoma); the second can be a lesion of undertermined malignant potential, for which the pathologist can not predict the biological behavior. The importance of recognizing these lesions hardly needs to be stated. Three recently described lesions that deserve to be briefly discussed are giant cell fibroblastoma [1], intranodal myofibroblastoma [2,3], and AIDS-associated pseudoangiomatous lesions [4]. Giant cell fibroblastoma is a tumor of children and most often is located in the trunk and thigh. Local recurrences occur in more than 50% of the cases mainly because of incomplete resection; metastases have not been reported. On microscopic examination, giant cell fibroblastoma is characterized by a combination of variable collagenized spindle cell and/or myxoid areas, pleomorphic, hyperchromatic, and multinucleated giant cells, and distinctive, virtually diagnostic sinusoid-like spaces. Mitoses are scarce and normal. Depending on the predominant pattern, the lesion may be confused with

Pinedo, H.M., Verweij, J., and H.D. Suit (eds.): Soft Tissue Sarcomas: New Developments in the Multidisciplinary Approach to Treatment. © 1991 Kluwer Academic Publishers, Boston. ISBN: 0–7923–1139–6. All rights reserved.

Table 1. Lesions that can be confused with high-grade sarcomas.

a. **Benign lesions mimicking sarcomas**
   Nodular fasciitis and related lesions
   Proliferative fasciitis and myositis
   Reactive histiocytosis
   Proliferative myositis
   Pleomorphic lipoma
   Lipoblastomatosis
   Papillary endothelial hyperplasia
   Radiation fibrosis
   Degenerating neurofibroma
   Cellular schwannoma
   Synovial chondromatosis
   Florid tendon sheath tumor with glandular spaces

b. **Tumors of borderline malignancy**
   Atypical fibroxanthoma
   Dermatofibrosarcoma protuberans
   Epithelial hemangioendothelioma
   Spindle cell hemangioendothelioma
   Papillary endovascular endothelioma
   Bednar tumor

malignant fibrous histiocytoma, myxoid liposarcoma, dermatofibrosarcoma protuberans, or angiosarcoma when prominent interstitial hemorrhage is present. The lack of atypical mitoses and lipoblasts and the rarity of such sarcomas in the juvenile population should prevent misdiagnoses. The histogenesis of giant cell fibroblastoma is still uncertain. A vascular origin has been ruled out. A fibroblastic and/or myofibroblastic nature of the cells is likely, and this tumor is included in the group of fibromatoses of childhood. Intranodal myofibroblastoma is a distinctive benign tumor of adults, which commonly occurs in lymph nodes of the groin [2,3], but may be seen elsewhere. It consists of short fascicles of spindle cells with wavy nuclei and focally nuclear palisading resembling neurilemoma; hence the term "palisaded myofibroblastoma". Mitoses are rare, and nuclear atypia virtually absent. Stellate areas of hyalinized collagen deposition, reported as "amianthoid" fibers with variable central calcification, are characteristic of this tumor. Interstitial hemorrhage frequently occurs, and a rim of recognizable nodal tissue is consistently found around the lesion. Treatment consists of simple excision; recurrences have not been reported. As benign spindle cell tumors occur very rarely in lymph nodes (i.e., neurofibroma, naevus cell inclusions, or benign vascular proliferations), the differential diagnosis of myofibroblastoma mainly includes Kaposi's sarcoma and metastatic spindle cell neoplasms, such as leiomyosarcoma, malignant fibrous histiocytoma, synovialosarcoma, spindle cell carcinoma, or melanoma. Before being individualized, intranodal myofibroblastomas were formerly classified as neurilemoma of the lymph node. However, immunohistochemical and ultrastructural studies have shown that tumor cells were not related to

2

Schwann's cell, but had features resembling that of myofibroblast. A benign cutaneous epithelioid vascular proliferation called "bacillary angiomatosis" has been described in patients with immunodeficiency syndrome. Clinically, they presented as multiple violaceous nodules mimicking Kaposi's sarcoma. On microscopic examination, they often show a distinctive lobular architecture resembling that of lobular capillary hemangioma or pyogenic granuloma. Atypical endothelial cells, with occasional mitoses and histiocytoides features as well as clumps of bacilli resembling cat scratch disease bacteria surrounded with acute inflammation and polymorphonuclear debris, are consistently found. The differential diagnosis includes Kaposi's sarcoma as well as epithelioid hemangioendothelioma, histiocytoid hemangioma, and the cutaneous lesion of Oraya fever. Reactive in their nature, these lesions respond to antibiotherapy. Another type of pseudosarcomatous spindle cell lesion related to nontuberculous mycobacteriosis has also been reported in lymph nodes and skin of patients with AIDS [5]. Florid proliferative tumors of the tendon sheath with pseudoglandular spaces can be misdiagnosed as synovial sarcoma. Nodules of lobular hemangioma can also show marked atypia and proliferative activity and be entirely benign. Pathologists should avoid considering these clearly and invariably benign lesions as "low-grade sarcomas" because they never progress. The biological hallmark of a low-grade malignant mesenchymal lesion is its capacity to progress. In this sense some, if not many, borderline lesions belonging to the group of undetermined malignant potential can be considered as low-grade sarcomas: lesions that will locally recur and eventually progress with metastases after several local recurrences. They can be treated with a conservative wide excision.

Immunohistochemistry and electron microscopy are widely used in most laboratories. Both contribute greatly to the classification of sarcomas [6], but immunohistochemistry has become the more widely used one. Immunochemistry justified diagnostic changes with therapeutic implications in 12% of the cases examined in the frame of a multicentric study of soft tissue sarcomas [7]. It is a technique of great value in the differential diagnosis between undifferentiated carcinoma, sarcoma, melanoma, and large cell lymphoma. The distinction relies mostly on the typing of the intermediate filaments expressed by the tumor cells. Malignant melanoma is undoubtedly the greatest mimicker. It can present as malignant fibrous histiocytoma, fibrosarcoma, or myxoid liposarcoma. Reactivity against Vimentin, S–100, NKI/C3, in an undifferentiated malignant tumor of soft parts should strongly suggest the possibility of melanoma, and electron microscopy should be done in order to conclusively establish the diagnosis. Kindblom has found premelanosomes in 21 out on 23 metastatic melanomas presenting as soft tissue mass. It is now well established that the tumor originally described as a "clear cell sarcoma" is a primary melanoma of the soft tissues and should be treated as such. When using intermediate filaments immunoreactivity to type tumors, it is important to keep in mind that "aberrant expression" is being described with increasing frequency. Cytokeratin-type filaments can

3

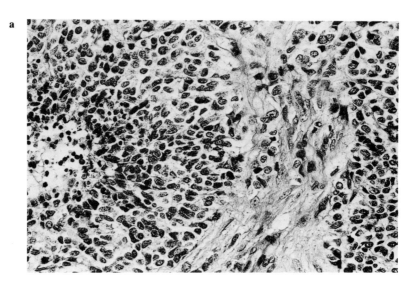

Figure 1. Examples of "differentiated" and "dedifferentiated" tumors. *Figure 1a.* Intra-abdominal mass of a young child with a desmoplastic small cell tumor. The tumor was positive for keratin, NSI, and desmin.

be detected in leiomyosarcomas [8], malignant fibrous histiocytomas [9], rhabdomyosarcomas [10], angiosarcomas [11], melanomas [12], astrocytomas [13], and neuroectodermal tumors [14]. Endothelial cells can also occasionally express cytokeratins. Aberrant expression of intermediate filaments underscores two important principles of the use of immunohistochemistry. First, a broad pannel of antisera should be used whenever possible; the use of one or two antisera, chosen to prove one's diagnosis, is dangerous. Second, positive staining should always be interpreted in the context of the gross and microscopic characteristics of the lesion. Reactivity in a small subpopulation of tumor cells should be interpreted with caution.

One of the contributions of immunocytochemistry is the capability to define the different cellular populations participating in the formation of a tumor mass. Supporting stromal cells, reactive cells (such as myofibroblasts or lymphoreticular cells), and distinct subpopulations of neoplastic cells can be distinguished by the expression of different antigenic determinants. Dramatic examples are multipartite tumors in which the cells differentiate along different pathways. The multipotentiality of the neoplastic cells of soft tissue tumors is clearly seen in childhood tumors. Some of the "round cell tumors" can remain undifferentiated or can show a mixed population of cells, some of which will exhibit neuronal characteristics, others a muscle phenotype, and yet others glial or melanocytic differentiation. Complex populations are seen in peripheral primitive neuroectodermal tumors and in "desmoplastic small cell tumors [15] (figure 1a). Such "primitive" or multipotential neoplasms can serve as models to learn about early mesenchymal

4

cell derivation. Preliminary reports suggest that cells derived from osteosarcoma can be transformed into contractile myotubes by transfection and
presumably expression of the MyoD-1 gene, a gene involved in early
myogenesis [16]. This work illustrates how mesenchymal cells can serve
as targets to assay a gene involved in early muscle differentiation. Another
study at the molecular level suggests that the *gli* oncogene, first discovered in gliomas, can influence gene expression in early mesenchymal
differentiation [17].

Opposite to the phenomenon of multipotentiality is "dedifferentiation".
This view has recently emerged from the observation that many different
types of sarcomas can show the histological characteristics of pleomorphic
malignant fibrous histiocytoma (PMFH). Evans was among the first to use
the term "dedifferentiated liposarcoma" by analogy to the "dedifferentiated
skeletal chondrosarcoma" [18]. Soft tissue chondrosarcoma, leiomyosarcoma, liposarcoma, and neurofibrosarcoma are among the histotypes
that can have areas indistinguishable from PMFH (figures 1b, 1c). With
progression, some of the tumors can lose the differentiated phenotype, but
immunochemistry can still show expression of a histotypic marker. As
there are no specific histiocytic antigenic markers, PMFH, as an entity
diagnosed by conventional histology, is likely to represent a mixture of
tumors derived from different cell types. It can be conceived as the common
end point of tumor progression for many malignant tumors of soft tissue.
Although the histogenesis of PMFH can be challenged, it remains a useful
clinicopathological entity.

Cytogenetic studies of soft tissue sarcomas have uncovered type-specific
alterations at the chromosomal level (Table 2). The interest of these abnor-
malities is that they point towards genetic loci that are likely to play a role in
the pathogenesis of these tumors and lead to the identification and isolation
of cancer genes operative in sarcomas. The advances in molecular diagnos-
tics make it very likely that the field of soft tissue tumors will benefit from
this approach in the near future, although at present these assays remain
entirely investigational. Candidate genes of interest include the retinoblastoma gene [19] and the p 53 gene [20].

The pathological study of tumors not only yields a diagnosis, but also
important prognostic information such as the adequacy of resection margins.
This requires also that the pathologist defines the orientation of the specimen at surgery and then determines the status of the margins with reference
to specific portions of the surgical field. Tumor grade is an accepted prognostic and staging parameter, but consensus as how to grade has not yet been
achieved. Can one grade across histotypes, or should grading be done only
within a histological type? The question is a difficult one.

Most of the grading systems that have been proposed discriminate three
of four prognostic groups among the sarcomas when disease free or overall
survival are used as endpoints [21,22,23]. We use a grading system that is
based on the NCI experience [24] and that is both based on the histological

5

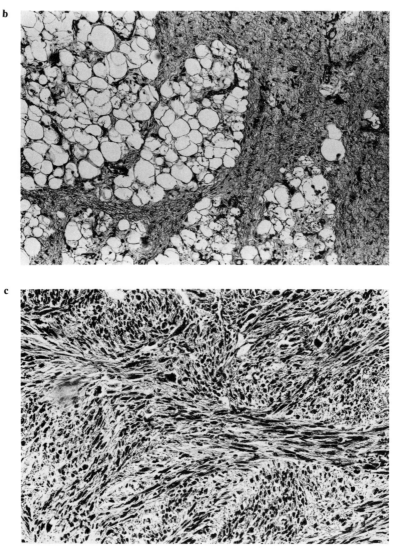

Figure 1b and 1c. Well-differentiated and sclerosing liposarcoma (1b) with extensive areas indistinguishable from pleomorphic MFH (1c).

type of the lesion and on histological features. The histological features used and their weight is in part modulated by the histotype. An updated description of the method has been given elsewhere [25].

Progress in grading can come, in two ways. One would be to carry out a multicentric study of well-characterized cases that are graded by different methods to try to come to a consensus. An alternative strategy is to attempt to find different approaches that can predict the biological behavior of a

Table 2. Chromosome and genetic alterations in soft tissue tumors.

Tumor	Chromosome	Reference
Peripheral neuroepithelioma	t (11;22)(q24;q12)	30
Synovial sarcoma	t (x;18) (p11;q12)	31
Alveolar rhabdomyosarcoma	t (2;13) (q37;q14)	32
Embryonal rhabdomyosarcoma	11p 15.5 11pter	33
Myxoid liposarcoma	t (12;16)(q13;p11)	34
Solitary lipomas	varied	35

given lesion (e.g., risk of metastasis), based on a different criteria than grade. Correlations of DNA content of the tumor cells (ploidy) with prognosis are of interest for a number of tumors. It is possible to think that ploidy profiles could contribute useful information at least for some histotypes of malignant soft tissue tumor. Interestingly, many of the malignant tumors that have been studied show no aneuploid DNA stem lines [26,27]. However, in MFH a possible correlation between aneuploidy and recurrence has been noted in at least one study [28]. Data should accumulate in the forthcoming years. Whether other morphometric methods can be used, such as suggested by Zeppa et al. in bone chondrosarcoma, remains to be demonstrated [29].

Another approach has been adopted by Perosio and Brooks. They investigate the expression of growth factors and their receptors in normal soft tissues and in a group of tumors. Their work suggests that coexpression of multiple growth factors and receptors is related to the biological potential among human soft tissue tumors [30]. One would hope that biochemical and molecular studies will contribute to our ability to predict the natural history of soft tissue sarcomas in the near future.

References

1. Shmookler BM, Enzinger FM, Weiss SW: Giant cell fibroblastoma. A juvenile form of dermatofibrosarcoma protuberans. Cancer 64:2154—2161, 1989.
2. Suster S, Rosai J: Intranodal hemorrhagic spindle-cell tumor with "amianthoid" fibers. Report of six cases of a distinctive mesenchymal neoplasm of the inguinal region that simulates Kaposi's sarcoma. Am J Surg Pathol 13:347—357, 1989.
3. Weiss SW, Gnepp DR, Bratthauer GL: Palisaded myofibroblastoma. A benign mesenchymal tumor of lymph node. Am J Surg Pathol 13:341—346, 1989.
4. Walford N, Van Der Wouw PA, Das PK, Ten Velden JJAM, Hulsebosch HJ: Epithelioid angiomatosis in the acquired immunodeficiency syndrome: Morphology and differential diagnosis. Histopathology 16:83—88, 1990.
5. Brandwein M, Choi HSH, Strauchen J, Stoler M, Jagirdar J: Spindle cell reaction to nontuberculous mycobacteriosis in AIDS mimicking a spindle cell neoplasm. Virchows Arch [A] 416:281—286, 1990.
6. Angervall L, Kindblom LG: The diagnosis of soft tissue tumors. The Göteborg experience.

In: Recent concepts in sarcoma treatment. Ryan J, Bahn LO, (eds). Boston: Kluwer Academic Publishers, pp 22—26, 1988.

7. Brooks JJ: Immunochemistry in sarcomas. In: Recent concepts in sarcoma treatment. Ryan J, Bahn LO, (eds). Boston: Kluwer Academic Publishers, pp 48—55, 1988.

8. Miettinen M: Immunoreactivity for cytokeratin and epithelial membrane antigen in leiomyosarcoma. Arch Pathol Lab Med 112:637—640, 1988.

9. Weiss SW, Brathauer GL, Morris PA: Postirradiation malignant fibrous histiocytoma expressing cytokeratin. Am J Surg Pathol 12:554—558, 1988.

10. Miettinen M, Rapola J: Immunohistochemical spectrum of rhabdomyosarcoma and rhabdomyosarcoma-like tumors. Expression of cytokeratin and the 68 kd neurofilament protein. Am J Surg Pathol 13:120—132, 1989.

11. Brooks JJ: Seminar on soft tissue pathology. European Society of Pathology, Porto, 1989.

12. Lambe CDK, Cartun RW, Knibbs DR, et al.: Immunocytochemical reactivity with cytokeratin monoclonal antibodies in malignant melanoma. Further evidence dictating cautious interpretation of immunostaining. Lab Invest 60:50a, 1989.

13. Costrove M, Fitzgibbons PL, Sherrod A, et al.: Intermediate filament expression in astrocytic neoplasms. Am J Surg Pathol 13:141—145, 1989.

14. Zarbo RJ, Raju U, Regezi J, et al.: Melanotic neuroectodermal tumors (MNT) of infancy: Intermediate filament, neuroendocrine and melanoma associated antigen profile. Lab Invest 60:109a, 1989.

15. Gerald W, Rosai J: Desmoplastic small cell tumor with divergent differentiation. Ped Pathol 9:177—183, 1989.

16. Chen J, Jones PA: Conversion of human osteogenic sarcoma cells into contractile myotubes by a muscle determination gene. Proc Am Assoc Cancer Res 30 (Abstr.):42, 1989.

17. Roberts WM, Douglas EC, Peiper S, et al.: Amplification of the gli gene in childhood sarcomas. Cancer Res 49:5407—5413, 1989.

18. Evans HL: Liposarcoma. A study of 55 cases with reassessment of its classification. Am J Surg Pathol 3:507, 1979.

19. Friend SH, Horowitz JM, Gerber M, et al.: Deletions of DNA sequence in retinoblastoma and mesenchymal tumors: Organization and sequence of the encoded protein. Proc Natl Acad Sci USA 84:9059—9063, 1987.

20. Chen H, Miller C, Koeffer HP, et al.: Rearrangement of the p 53 gene in human osteogenic sarcomas. Proc Natl Acad Sci USA 84:7716—7719, 1987. Perosio MP, Brooks JJ: Expression of growth factors and growth factor receptors in soft tissue tumors. Lab Invest 60:245—253, 1989.

21. Markhede G, Angervall L, Stener B: A multivariate analysis of the prognosis after surgical treatment of malignant soft tissue tumors. Cancer 49:1721—1723, 1982.

22. Trojani M, Contesso G, Coindre JM, et al.: Soft tissue sarcoma of the adults: Study of pathological prognostic variables and definition of histopathological grading system. Int J Cancer 33:37—42, 1983.

23. Mandard AM, Petiot J, Marnay J, et al.: Prognostic factors in soft tissue sarcomas. A multivariate analysis (109 cases). Cancer 63:1437—1451, 1989.

24. Costa J, Wesley RA, Glatstein E, et al.: The grading of soft tissue sarcomas: Results of a clinico-histopathological correlation in a series of 163 cases. Cancer 53:530—541, 1984.

25. Leyvraz S, Costa J: Histological diagnosis and grading of soft tissue sarcomas. Semin Surg Oncol 4:3—6, 1988.

26. Kreicbergs A, Tribukait B, Willems J, et al.: DNA flow analysis of soft tissue tumors. Cancer 59:128—133, 1987.

27. Schmidt D, Leuschner I, Harms D, et al.: Malignant rhabdoid tumor. A morphological and flow cytometric study. Pathol Res Pract 184:202—210, 1989.

28. Radio SJ, Wooldridge I, Linder J: Flow cytometry DNA analysis of malignant fibrous histiocytoma and related fibrohistiocytic tumors. Human Pathol 19:74—77, 1988.

29. Zeppa P, Zabatta A, Marino G, et al.: A morphometric approach to the grading of chondroid tumors on fine-needle smears. Pathol Res Pract 185:760—763, 1989.

30. Turc–Carel C, Lizard–Nacol S, Justrabo E, et al.: Two new cases of primary peripheral neuroepithelioma of soft tissue with translocation T (11;22) (Q24;Q12). Cancer genet Cytogenet 33:291—297, 1988.
31. Turc–Carel C, Dal Cin P, Limon J, et al.: Translocation X:18 in synovial sarcoma. Cancer Genet Cytogenet 23:93, 1986.
32. Turc–Carel C. Lizard–Nacol S, Justrabo E, et al.: Consistant chromosome translocation in alveolar rhabdomyosarcoma. Cancer Genet Cytogenet 19:361—362, 1986.
33. Scrable HJ, Lamplin BC, Witte OP, et al.: Mitotic recombination mapping localizes the human rhabdomyosarcoma locus to chromosome 11p 15.5 11pter. Nature 329:645—647, 1987.
34. Turc–Carel C, Limon J, Dal Cin P, et al.: Cytogenetic studies of adipous tissue tumors. Cancer Genet Cytogenet 23:291—299, 1986.
35. Mandahl N, Heim S, Arheden K, et al.: Three major cytogenetic subgroups can be identified among chromosomally abnormal solitary lipomas. Human Genet 79:203—208, 1988.

2. Diagnostic Imaging

Holger Pettersson and Kristian Herrlin

Introduction

During the last decades, the clinical approach to soft tissue sarcomas has changed considerably, from amputation towards limb-salvage surgery, without adverse effects on patient survival or limb function [1]. Such procedures are possible only after precise preoperative evaluation of the local extent of the lesion, and this evaluation demands modern diagnostic imaging.

Parallel with the development of new treatment approaches, the different diagnostic imaging modalities have improved. As a matter of fact, the improvements in diagnostic imaging have been an important basis for the improvement of treatment. Today, plain film radiography, angiography, bone scintigraphy, ultrasound (US), computed tomography (CT), and magnetic resonance imaging (MRI) are the diagnostic tools that may be used in the evaluation of any tumor. In this chapter, we will discuss the state of the art of diagnostic imaging of soft tissue sarcomas, comparing the possibilities and limitations provided by the different modalities.

Diagnostic Imaging Approach to Soft Tissue Sarcomas

It should be stressed that radiologic evaluation is part of a team work [2]. The radiologic evaluation is an integral part of the total assessment of the patient, and the final decisions should be made within the treatment team. The goal of the radiologic investigations should be
1. To evaluate the aggressiveness and possible diagnosis of the tumor, which is important information for the decision on further management of the patient. Such assessment is more important for bone tumors than for soft tissue tumors, as most deep-seated (below the fascia) soft tissue tumors should be regarded as aggressive and possibly malignant.
2. To define in great detail the local extent of the tumor.

For adequate diagnostic imaging work-up, good equipment and a proper technique are mandatory. We will therefore first discuss the imaging technique, and after that, the evaluation of soft tissue tumors with different types of diagnostic imaging modalities.

Pinedo, H.M., Verweij, J., and H.D. Suit (eds.): Soft Tissue Sarcomas: New Developments in the Multidisciplinary Approach to Treatment. © *1991 Kluwer Academic Publishers, Boston. ISBN: 0–7923–1139–6. All rights reserved.*

Imaging Techniques

Conventional Radiography

Plain film radiography is often used as the first radiologic evaluation of the tumor, but for soft tissue tumors, its value is limited. Occasionally, calcifications may be seen in a vascular tumor, and seldom bone erosion caused by a soft tissue tumor may be detected. However, conventional radiographs do provide a convenient baseline for the evaluation of the status of the bone following drug and radiation therapy.

Angiography

Angiography was for a long time indispensable for the assessment of soft tissue sarcomas [3]. However, with modern CT equipment and more recently with MRI, the indications for angiography have diminished considerably.

The technique does not differ significantly from other diagnostic angiographic examinations. Small catheters (4 to 5 F) have become increasingly common. For leg examinations, the contralateral femoral artery should be punctured, and the catheter should be fed over the aortic bifurcation down to the side of the lesion. For arm lesions, the brachial or femoral approach may be used.

Digital subtraction angiography (DSA) enables the use of even smaller catheters. Although the spatial resolution with this technique is not as good as with film-screen combinations, the tumor blush of vascular tumors is usually better, and the venous phase is also excellent [4].

Ultrasonography

This method has become common for the evaluation of several orthopedic lesions, but for soft tissue sarcomas the value is limited. Although solid and cystic soft tissue masses can be differentiated, the local behavior of a tumor cannot be assessed, and there is little information as to the diagnosis [5].

Scintigraphy

Scintigraphy, is yet of limited value. Bone scintigraphy, using 99m-Tc, sometimes indicates an uptake of the isotope in the primary tumor [6]. Also, scintigraphy using 67-Ga has sometimes resulted in uptake by soft tissue tumors [7]. If whole-body images are obtained routinely, a spot film of the diseased area is important. With modern detection systems, the entire examination may be performed with spot films of different anatomic areas, and then the sum of the spot areas should cover the whole body.

Specific tumor seeking agents in the form of isotope-labeled monoclonal antibodies are under development. As yet, they have no established role in the diagnosis of soft tissue sarcomas, but early reports are promising [8].

Computed Tomography (CT)

The introduction of CT in the diagnostic imaging arsenal meant a revolution, mainly for three reasons:
1. The much better contrast resolution compared with the previously used methods.
2. The ability to provide cross-sectional imaging.
3. The possibility for tissue differentiation and characterization, measuring the attenuation values.

To perform an adequate CT examination, the following parameters must be set: scan volume (upper and lower limits), slice thickness and interval, reconstruction algorithm, field of view, and the use of oral and/or intravenous contrast medium. To get optimal information, the technique for image evaluation must also be considered.

Scan Volume   All modern scanners have equipment for digital radiography (scout view), and such an image must be obtained to define the proximal and distal points of the examination. Enough normal tissue on both sides of the tumor should be included to ensure that the entire tumor is examined. A plastic catheter placed over a scar or a palpable mass will be visible on the digitalized radiograph and may be helpful for localization.

Slice Thickness and Interval   The choice of slice thickness is mainly determined by the size of the tumor that is examined. However, there should be at least three sections through the lesion in order to minimize the effect of volume averaging. Also, the complexity of the neighboring anatomic structures should be considered.

However, the use of thin sections may lead to a large number of CT slices, prolonging the examination and increasing the radiation dose. Then thinner and thicker slices may be combined. As a rule the most complex anatomic information will be seen at the belly of an elliptic tumor and at the end and belly of a teardrop tumor, and in these areas thinner slices should be used. The CT sections should usually be obtained immediately adjacent to each other.

Reconstruction Algorithm   Most modern CT equipment provides options for several imaging algorithms. For evaluation of soft tissue tumors, it may be wise to obtain hard film copies, using not only soft tissue window for the evaluation of tumor contents and relation to neighboring soft tissues, but also bone window for the evaluation of the relation between the tumor and neighboring bone.

Field of View   The field of view (FOV) is the diameter of the reconstruction circle used by the CT computer to generate the film image. Reducing the FOV decreases the pixel size, leading to increased spatial resolution. Today with varying FOVs, the pixel size may range between 0.2 and 1 mm. However, even if a small FOV increases the spatial resolution, at the same time it excludes the opposite normal side of the body from comparison, and such comparison may be helpful in detecting subtle soft tissue changes. Also, a small FOV may decrease the contrast resolution. Therefore, a combination of FOVs may be a good compromise.

Oral and Intravenous Contrast Media   Musculoskeletal tumors should be examined both prior to i.v. contrast medium administration and during contrast medium infusion or after contrast medium bolus injection. The examination performed before contrast medium administration will reveal, for instance, calcifications in the tumor, and a comparison of the images obtained before and after contrast medium reveals tumor as well as the relation between the tumor and neighboring large vessels [9]. Oral contrast medium outlining the bowel is of importance for the evaluation of pelvic tumors, for instance.

Magnetic Resonance Imaging (MRI)

MRI has proven to be well suited for the examination of soft tissue tumors because of the high soft tissue resolution, the ease with which imaging in any plane may be performed, and the possibilities (although so far limited) for tissue characterization. However, MRI is a complex imaging modality requiring careful selection of several technical parameters in order to obtain optimal imaging. Such parameters include pulse sequences, coil selection, slice thickness, scan axis, and field of view. Also, the use of intravenous MR contrast media should be discussed.

Pulse Sequences   During the last years, the most widely utilized pulse sequence has been the spin-echo. Manipulating with the TR and TE of this sequence, a T1- or T2-weighted image may be obtained. A short TR (less than 500 msec) and short TE (less than 30 msec) provide a T1-weighted image, while a long TR-(more than 1,500 msec) and TE-(more than 40 msec) sequence is T2 weighted. For most soft tissue tumors, the tumor and muscle often have similar signal intensity in the T1-weighted image, while better tumor-muscle contrast is obtained in the T2-weighted image. In such images, the tumor has a high signal intensity. On the other hand, the distinction between tumor and fat may be poor in a T2-weighted image. Therefore, it has been common to perform both T1-weighted and a T2-weighted sequences for the evaluation of musculoskeletal tumors [10].

14

Three-dimensional (3-D) spin-echo technique may be helpful for determining the tumor extent in anatomically complex regions: for instance, invasion of the joints. The possible choices of pulse sequences are theoretically unlimited, and recently several new pulse sequence techniques have been proposed. The sequence that probably will, at least in part, replace the spin-echo imaging is the technique using reduced flip angles with gradient echoes. This technique allows image acquisition in much less time, reducing the motion artifacts, which is of interest for increasing patient through-put. It is also important for "dynamic imaging" in connection with MR intravenous contrast media [11].

Coil Selection   All modern MR units offer not only standard "body coils", but also smaller specialized receiver coils. These specialized coils improve the image quality by (1) increasing the signal strength received from a patient; and (2) reducing the volume of irradiated tissue covered by the coil, thus reducing the image noise [12]. Depending on the MR equipment, the design of the coils will vary, but generally, specialized receiver coils designed for different anatomic areas should be used for the imaging of musculoskeletal tumors.

Slice Thickness   In most patients a slice thickness varying between 4 to 10 mm is appropriate. Using spin-echo imaging, contigous slices are not possible to obtain. Theoretically, gaps between the slices may mean that important information could be missed. However, for most MR images available today, the interslice gap is relatively small and should not create a practical problem.

Field of View   The field of view is defined as the diameter of the scan field on which the image matrix is applied. Reducing the field of view increases the spatial resolution, but may also decrease the signal intensity. A reduced field of view is recommended for the distal extremities and anatomic details. A proper balance between the field of view and degradation of the image quality must be determined for each type of equipment.

Tissue Characterization   MR provides high soft tissue contrast discrimination. The contrast in the image is mainly determined by T1 and T2 characteristics of the tissue, the proton density, and flow. It is also dependant on the pulse sequences used. As different tissues have different T1 and T2 values, the relative contribution of the T1 and T2 to the image contrast may be altered by manipulation of the pulsing sequence. Then, comparing T1- and T2-weighted images may allow tissue characterization.

Concerning the normal bone and soft tissues, muscle and articular cartilage usually have an intermediate signal intensity both in the T1- and T2-weighted images, except in strongly T2-weighted images where they become dark. Cortical bones are dark (low signal intensity) in all sequences, and fat is very bright in all sequences.

Most tumors have a prolonged T1 and T2 as compared to muscle and fat. On T1-weighted spin-echo images, tumors usually have the same signal intensity as muscle, but are darker than fat. On the T2-weighted images, the tumors become brighter than muscle, and on strongly T2-weighted images, tumors usually also become brighter than fat [13].

Much MR equipment today provides possibilities for the calculation of exact T1 and T2 values. However, these values depend both on imaging technique and field strength, and as a whole, the exact T1 and T2 values for tissue characterization have proven to be of little importance, as will be discussed below [15,16].

Intravenous Contrast Media Today the most frequently used intravenous MR contrast medium is based on Gadolinium (Gadolinium-DTPA/Gd-DTPA or Gadolinium-DOTA/Gd-DOTA). Being administered intravenously, it is distributed in accordance with traditional intravenous contrast media used in radiology, giving information on vascular permeability and increased blood flow. Therefore, it may be of value both for the assessment of the vascularization of the tumor and for detailed evaluation of its local extent (see below) [11,16].

Evaluation of Soft Tissue Tumors

As stated above, the radiologic evaluation of soft tissue tumors should include (1) an assessment of local aggressiveness, (2) a probable diagnosis, (3) the local extent of the tumor, and (4) possible involvement of adjacent bone.

Aggressiveness

For the assessment of the aggressiveness of soft tissue tumors, all diagnostic imaging modalities are of limited value. Conventional radiographs rarely provide any information. Bone scintigraphy may give rough information on the aggressiveness, since aggressive lesions have a considerably increased uptake, while slow growing lesions may have slight or no uptake at all [6]. At angiography, there is a good correlation between the degree of pathologic vascularization and the differentiation of the tumor, but angiographically, avascular masses may also be highly malignant [17]. MRI as well as CT are of limited value for the evaluation of the aggressiveness of soft tissue tumors. As a whole, there are no methods that significantly contribute to the evaluation of the aggressiveness. Therefore, with the exception of lipoma (see below), all deep soft tissue tumors should be approached as if they were aggressive [18].

16

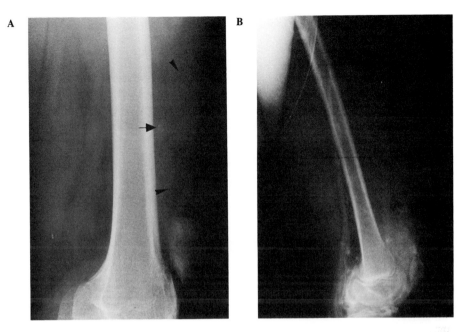

Figure 1. Radiologic patterns, plain film radiography, and angiography. Cavernous hemangioma. (A) There is a singular calcification (black arrow) and a tortuous structure (arrowheads) in the anterior portion of the thigh, suggestive of distended vessels. (B) Arteriography. In the capillary phase there is contrast filling of a cavernous hemangioma.

Diagnosis

In establishing the diagnosis of a soft tissue tumor, the aggressiveness of the tumor, its location, the possible multiplicity of the tumor, and specific radiologic patterns of the tumor matrix must be determined. To this, several important clinical data should be added: the age of the patient, the history, findings at clinical examination, laboratory data, etc. To obtain this information, different combinations of the diagnostic imaging modalities have been used.

Plain film examinations yield little diagnostic information. However, calcified phlebolites may be seen in a tumor of vascular origin (figure 1a), and a low density of a lipoma may be recognized [19].

Ultrasound may be used for differentiation between solid and cystic lesions, but the greatest value of ultrasound is to serve as a guide for the biopsy of soft tissue tumors (figure 2) [20].

Scintigraphy is an excellent tool for the evaluation of multiplicity of a lesion. Otherwise, the information gained from scintigraphy is nonspecific for the diagnosis [21].

The diagnostic capability of angiography is limited. Vascular tumors, such as angiolipoma and cavernous venous hemangioma, can be diagnosed at

17

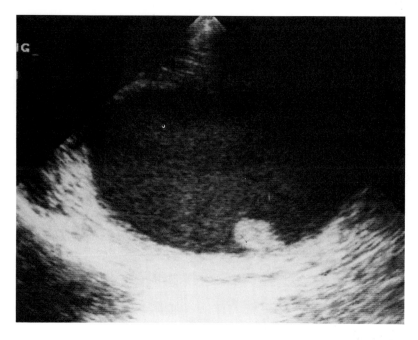

Figure 2. Ultrasound as a guide for biopsy. Malignant fibrous histiocytoma. At ultrasound examination, a tumor nodule is seen adjacent to the capsule. The central area of homogenous echogenicity represents a large hematoma. If biopsy is performed, it should be directed towards the tumor nodule in the periphery.

angiographic examination (figure 1b), but the overlap between different tumor types is considerable.

Occasionally, CT may reveal clues that lead to a tissue diagnosis. This especially concerns vascular tumors and lipomas (figure 3). If a tumor is homogenous, with a density varying between-60 and 100-Hounsfield units, the diagnosis of a lipoma is certain [22]. Otherwise, the density of soft tissue tumors is not useful for distinguishing benign from malignant lesions. However, malignant soft tissue tumors tend to be more inhomogeneous, involve multiple muscles, have irregular borders, and blurr the adjacent fat, while benign lesions tend to be homogeneous, involve only one muscle, and do not blurr adjacent fat [9]. But in the individual case, CT will not be reliable for distinguishing malignant from benign lesions (figure 4). CT may also be helpful in guiding biopsy or aspiration of bone or soft tissue tumors (figure 5).

On MR images, most musculoskeletal tumors have a similar appearance: low signal intensity (dark, about the same as muscle) on T1-weighted spin-echo images, and high signal intensity (white) on T2-weighted images (figure 6). Exceptions to this pattern exist, and such exceptions may be a clue to diagnosis. Tumors with high signal intensity both on T1- and T2-weighted images may contain fat, hemorrhage, or slowly flowing blood. Conversely,

18

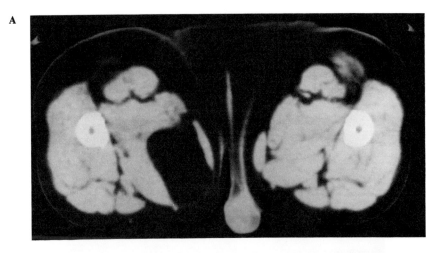

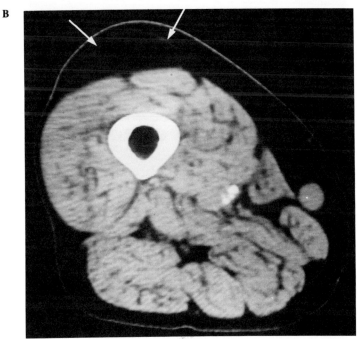

Figure 3. CT pattern; soft tissue lipoma. (A) Intramuscular lipoma, right thigh. Note the homogenous density of the lesion similar to the density of the subcutaneous fat. (B) Sub-cutaneous lipoma anteriorly in the thigh. In this location lipomas are less clearly seen, being isodense with the surrounding fat. A thin capsule surrounds the lipoma (arrows).

19

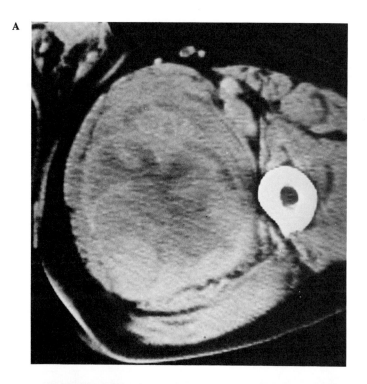

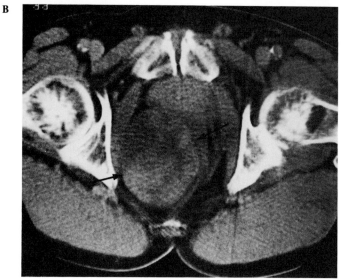

Figure 4. Two different types of soft tissue tumors with similar pattern at CT. (A) Malignant fibrous histiocytoma in the abductor magnus muscle of the thigh. Note the irregular enhancement after contrast administration, suggestive of central necrosis. (B) Perineal angioleiomyoma — a benign smooth muscle tumor (arrows). The internal structure is similar to that of the lesion in (A). In both cases the irregular contrast enhancement reflects the uneven vascular supply to the tumor.

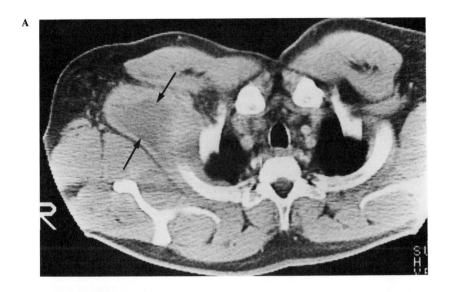

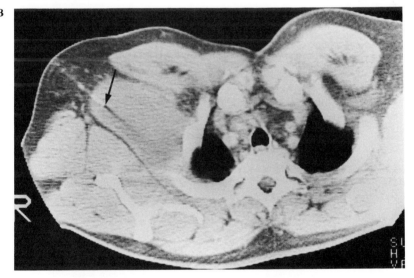

Figure 5. CT as guide for biopsy; malignant fibrous histiocytoma, right chest wall. (A) At CT with contrast enhancement, a hypolucent area is seen in the central portion of the tumor, suggestive of fluid or necrosis (arrows). (B) With knowledge of the internal structure of the lesion above, at subsequent CT-guided fine-needle biopsy, the puncture is performed in the border zone between enhanced and nonenhanced tissue (arrow).

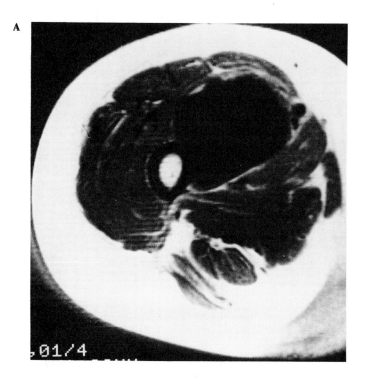

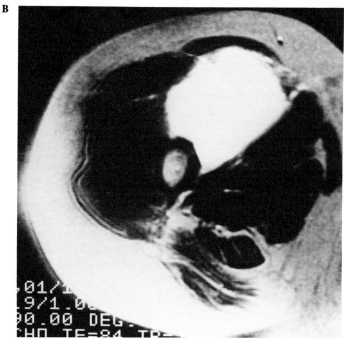

Figure 6. MR appearance of soft tissue tumor MRI of a myxoid fibrosarcoma grade I of the vastus medialis muscle. (A) A T1-weighted spin-echo sequence. The whole tumor has a low signal intensity. (B) T2-weighted spin-echo sequence. In this sequence the tumor has a high signal intensity, providing excellent contrast with the bone and surrounding muscles.

lesions with low signal intensity on the T2-weighted images are probably acellular and contain mostly collagen, are calcified, or have a rapid blood flow. MRI has a low capability of detecting calcifications [23].

Although some authors have reported malignant tumors to be more commonly inhomogeneous with irregular, poorly defined margins, there are many exceptions to this general rule [24].

Recently, dynamic Gd-DTPA-enhanced MR imaging using fast low angle shot (FLASH) sequences have been reported to be useful, giving information about the malignant potential of a tumor, although with certain overlap between benign and malignant tumors [11].

However, there are some specific MR patterns that may provide a clue to the diagnosis: if a tumor has the same high signal intensity as the subcutaneous fat both in the T1- and T2-weighted images, it is very probably a lipoma. However, a lipoma may be difficult to distinguish at MRI from a hematoma of intermediate age. Also, subcutaneous lipomas can have a very thin capsule that may not be visible on MR, and therefore, it may not be possible to distinguish the tumor from the surrounding fat. Although the T1 and T2 values of the tumor tissue may be calculated in each patient, there is growing experience that such values are of little or no value for suggesting a specific histopathologic diagnosis [15,16].

Local Extent of the Tumor

Evaluation of the local extent of the tumor is of utmost importance for the preoperative planning. For this planning as well as for purposes of surgical staging, the extremities are considered to be divided into various anatomic compartments [25].

A compartment is an anatomic structure surrounded by natural barriers for tumor growth. Such barriers are the cortical bone and the periosteum, the epiphyseal plate, and the articular as well as the epiphyseal cartilage. In soft tissue, the muscle fascia is a barrier towards tumor growth. Therefore, each bone is considered a compartment, as are the major muscle groups. Also, an isolated muscle may be considered a compartment. Certain regions of the body have no natural barriers to tumor growth and are consequently classified as primary extracompartmental anatomic sites.

An important goal with the evaluation of the local extent is to identify the compartment of origin, to depict the extent of a tumor within the compartment, and to note if the lesion has escaped this compartment. Also, it is important to evaluate the relation between the tumor and neighboring large vessels and nerves as well as bone.

CT is a good method for identifying the compartment of origin and the possible extension outside this compartment (figure 5) [26,27]. However, some tumors may be isodense with the muscle, making the detection difficult or impossible, and peritumoral edema and inflammatory reaction around the tumor may blurr adjacent soft tissue planes and lead to over-estimation of the tumor size [9,28] (figure 7a). Even if the intravenous contrast medium may improve the tumor visibility, CT is inferior to MR.

MRI is an excellent method for imaging soft tissue tumors because of its high soft tissue contrast resolution. There is no doubt that MRI today is far superior to any other method in defining the extent of soft tissue sarcoma (figure 7b) [13,14,23,29-31]. However, in certain cases it may be impossible to differentiate exactly between peritumoral edema, inflammatory reaction, and tumor, using SE-sequences (figure 8). For better differentiation, the use of intravenous Gadolinium-DTPA has been tried (figure 9). With traditional SE-sequences, the use of Gadolinium-DTPA seems only to reveal the vascularization of the tumor and of the peritumoral zone, giving no additional information on the differentiation between these structures [11,16]. However, dynamic studies urging FLASH-gradient-echo sequences may aid in the differentiation between tumor, edema, and normal tissue, as the edema has a slower gradual increase in signal intensity than the tumor [11].

Evaluation of the involvement of the great vessels and nerves is crucial, as this may determine if limb-salvage procedure is possible or not. At CT, involvement of the neurovascular bundle is detected in most cases. For such evaluation, intravenous contrast medium should be administered, preferably as a bolus. This is especially important when small vessels are imaged [2].

MRI is superior to other imaging modalities, because the contrast between the tumor and the vessels is generally high [13,14,16]. Also, the possibility of imaging longitudinal sections may add information concerning the relationship between the tumor and the neurovascular bundle.

Involvement of Adjacent Bone

Scintigraphy is rarely useful for the evaluation of bone involvement, but sometimes there is an uptake of the radionuclide both in the bone and the soft tissue tumor. Increased bone uptake, or direct continuity between tumor uptake and the bone, is considered positive for bone involvement, whereas normal uptake between the tumor and the bone is negative [32]. The value of CT is limited when the tumor is situated very near the bone, but not invading it. Here beam-hardening artifacts can interfere with the determination, as can the false "widening" of bone on soft tissue window settings.

MRI is an accurate method for delineation of the tumor/bone relationship [23]. If there is a sheet of normal tissue between the tumor and the bone, the bone is obviously not involved, and there is cortical bone invasion when there is a tumor signal seen within the normal cortex that normally has no signal. However, subtle invasion may be difficult to detect with MRI. ▶

Figure 7. Local extent, CT, and MRI; malignant fibrous histiocytoma, right thigh. (A) CT examination through the vertex of the lesion without contrast enhancement. A rather ill-defined soft tissue mass is seen in the vastus intermedius muscle. (B) T2-weighted spin-echo sequence, sagittal section. With this imaging sequence, optimal delineation of the tumor is achieved.

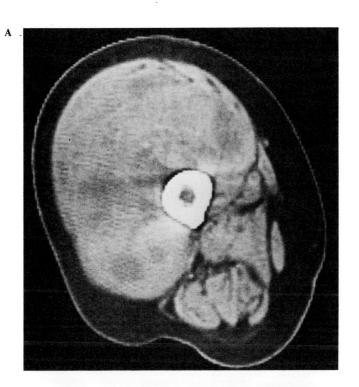

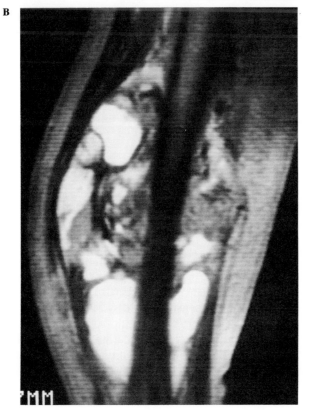

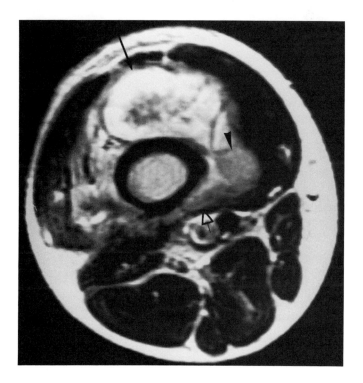

Figure 8. Difficulties in differentiation between tumor, peritumoral edema/inflammatory reaction, and normal tissue. Malignant fibrous histiocytoma right vastus intermedius muscle. T2-weighted spin-echo sequence. A tumor with high signal intensity is seen corresponding to the vastus intermedius muscle (arrow). In adjacent portions of the vastus medialis and lateralis, a diffuse area of intermediate signal intensity is seen (open arrow), which at surgery were found to represent edema. However, the round area of intermediate signal intensity on the medial side (arrowhead) represents tumor.

Conclusion

The successive advent of new imaging modalities has meant a dramatic improvement in the radiologic evaluation of musculoskeletal tumors and among those, also of soft tissue sarcomas. During the last years, several controlled studies have been published on the accuracy of the different imaging modalities, and there is a consensus tha MRI is superior in all important aspects for the evaluation of soft tissue tumors. Even if a combination of other methods may give acceptable and accurate results, MRI may well be used as the only diagnostic imaging modality in the evaluation of these lesions [14,16,29,30].

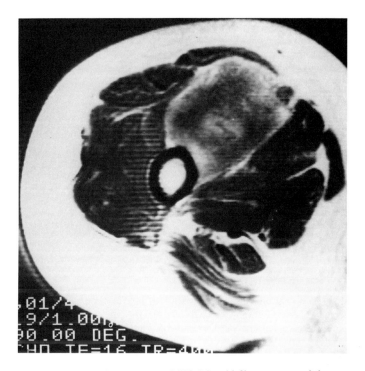

Figure 9. Contrast medium enhancement at MRI. Myxoid fibrosarcoma of the vastus medialis muscle; same patient as in figure 6. Following intravenous administration of Gd-DTPA, there is irregular enhancement of the tumor in the T1-weighted images corresponding to the vascularized strands of fibrous tissue within the tumor. The myxomatous parts of the tumor are not enhanced.

References

1. Sundaram M, McGuire MH, Herbold DR, Wolverson MK, Heiberg E: Magnetic resonance imaging in planning limb salvage surgery for primary malignant tumors of bone. J Bone Joint Surg (Am) 68:809—819, 1986.
2. Pettersson H, Springfield DS, Enneking WF: Radiologic management of musculoskeletal tumors. Berlin-Heidelberg: Springer–Verlag, 1987.
3. Hudson TM, Enneking WF, Hawkins IF, Jr: Value of angiography in planning surgical treatment of bone tumors. Radiology 138:283—292, 1981.
4. Hawkins IF: Angiography. In: Radiologic management of musculoskeletal tumors. Pettersson et al. (eds). Berlin-Heidelberg: Springer–Verlag: pp 21—26, 1987.
5. Scheible W: Diagnostic ultrasound. In: Diagnosis of bone and joint disorders. Resnick D, Niwayama G (eds). Philadelphia: WB Saunders, pp 409—421, 1981.
6. Chew FS, Hudson TM: Radionuclide imaging of lipoma and liposarcoma. Radiology 136:741—745, 1980.
7. Kirchner PT, Simon MA: The clinical value of bone and gallium scintigraphy for soft-tissue sarcomas of the extremities. J Bone Joint Surg (Am) 66:319—327, 1984.
8. Cox PH, Verweij J, Pillay M, Stoter G, Schonfeld D: Indium-111 antimyosin for the detection of leiomyosarcoma and rhabdomyosarcoma. Eur J Nucl Med 14:50—52, 1988.

9. Ekelund L, Herrlin K, Rydholm A: Comparison of computed tomography and angiography in the evaluation of soft tissue tumors of the extremities. Acta Radiol 23:15—28, 1982.

10. Richardson ML, Amparo EG, Gillespy T, III, Helms CA, Demas BE, Genant HK: Theoretical considerations for optimizing intensity differences between primary musculoskeletal tumors and normal tissue with spin-echo magnetic resonance imaging. Invest Radiol 20:492, 1985.

11. Erlemann R, Reiser MF, Peters PE, Vasallo P, Nommensen B, Kusnierz-Glaz CR, Ritter J, Roessner A: Musculoskeletal neoplasms: Static and dynamic Gd-DTPA-enhanced MR imaging. Radiology 171:767—773, 1989.

12. Kneeland JB, Hyde JS: High-resolution MR imaging with local coils. Radiology 171:1—7, 1989.

13. Pettersson H, Gillespy T, III, Hamlin DJ, Enneking WF, Springfield DS, Andrew R, Spanier S, Slone R: Primary musculoskeletal tumors: Examination with MR imaging compared with conventional modalities. Radiology 164:237—241, 1987.

14. Pettersson H, Eliasson J, Egund N. Rööser B, Willén H, Rydholm A, Berg NO, Holtås S: Gadolinium-DTPA enhancement of soft tissue tumors in magnetic resonance imaging — preliminary clinical experience in five patients. Skeletal Radiol 17:319—323, 1988.

15. Zimmer WD, Berquist TII, McLeod RA, et al.: Bone tumors: Magnetic resonance imaging versus computed tomography. Radiology 155:709—718, 1985.

16. Pettersson H, Slone RM, Spanier S, Gillespy T, III, Fitzsimmons JR, Scott, KN: Musculoskeletal tumors: T1 and T2 relaxation times. Radiology 167:783—785, 1988.

17. Hudson TM, Haas G, Enneking WF, Hawkins IF, Jr: Angiography in the management of musculoskeletal tumors. Surg Gynecol Obstet 141:11—21, 1975.

18. Rydholm A, Alvegård T, Berg NO, Dawiskiba Z, Egund N, Idvall I, Pettersson H, Rööser B, Willén H, Åkerman M: Preoperative diagnosis of soft tissue tumors. International Orthopaedics (SICOT) 12:109—114, 1988.

19. Hudson TM: Radiologic-pathologic correlation of musculoskeletal lesions. Baltimore: Williams and Wilkins, 1986.

20. Holm HH, Pedersen JF, Kristensen JK, Rasmussen SN, Hancke S, Jensen F: Ultrasonically guided percutaneous puncture. Radiol Clin North Am 13:493, 1975.

21. Springfield DS, Enneking WF, Neff JR, Mahley JT: Principles of tumor management: In: AAOS instructional course lectures. Murray JA (ed). St. Louis: CV Mosby, pp 1—24, 1984.

22. Hunter JC, Johnston WH, Genant HK: Computed tomography evaluation of fatty tumors of the somatic soft tissues: Clinical utility and radiologic–pathologic correlation. Skeletal Radiol 4:79—91, 1979.

23. Ehman RL, Berquist T, McLeod RA: MR imaging of the musculoskeletal system: A 5-year appraisal. Radiology 166:313—320, 1988.

24. Berquist TH: Bone and soft tissue tumors. In: Magnetic resonance of the musculoskeletal system. Berquist TH, Ehman RL, Richardson ML (eds). New York, Raven Press: pp 85—108, 1987.

25. Springfield DS: Surgical staging system. In: Radiologic management of musculoskeletal tumors. Pettersson H et al. (eds). Berlin–Heidelberg: Springer–Verlag, pp 5—6, 1987.

26. Rosenthal DI: Computed tomography in bone and soft tissue neoplasm: Application and pathologic correlation. CRC Crit Rev Diagn Imaging 18: 243—277, 1982.

27. Rosenthal DI: Computed tomography of orthopedic neoplasms. Orthop Clin North Am 16:461—470, 1985.

28. Egund N, Ekelund L, Sako M, Persson B: CT of soft-tissue tumors. AJR 137:725—729, 1981.

29. Demas BE, Heelan RT, Lane J, Marcove R, Hajdu S, Brennan MP: Soft-tissue sarcomas of the extremities: Comparison of MRI and CT in determining the extent of disease. AJR 150:615—620, 1988.

30. Sundaram M, McGuire MH, Herbold DR: Magnetic resonance imaging of soft tissue

masses: An evaluation of fifty-three histologically proven tumors. Magn Reson Imaging 6:237—248, 1988.

31. Tehranzadeh J, Mnaymneh W, Ghavam C, Morillo G, Murphy BJ: Comparison of CT and MR imaging in musculoskeletal neoplasms. J Comput Assist Tomogr 13:466—472, 1989.

32. Hudson TM, Schakel M, Springfield DS, Spanier SS, Enneking WF: The comparative value of bone scintigraphy and computed tomography in determining bone involvement by soft tissue sarcomas. J Bone Joint Surg (Am) 66:1400—1407, 1984.

3. Staging Soft Tissue Sarcomas

William O. Russell

The advances made over the past two decades in multimodal treatment for soft parts sarcoma with increased disease-free survival are among the notables in oncology achievements. More precise identification of tumor types, with better understanding of their biological behavior and therapeutic sensitivities, and the advances in diagnostic technology for assessment of the extent of disease have contributed to the maximum impact of the new, sophisticated uses and applications of surgery and radiation with the available chemical and immunobiological therapies.

Contributing to this concert application of these impacting advances in sarcoma treatment, TNM classification and staging of tumors has provided useful perspective information in the selection of a therapy, the determination of its intensity, and the extent of its application. Moreover, cancer staging assists the production of quality-controlled data to evaluate the effect of the therapies and the patient's survival for end-results reporting.

This chapter presents the soft tissue sarcoma staging system of the American Joint Committee on Cancer (AJCC) [1]. In 1986, the AJCC and the Union Internationale Contre le Cancer (UICC) TNM Committee reached principle, letter, and symbol agreement of their respective classifications for staging, thus establishing a worldwide agreement on the staging of cancer [2]. The staging system is designed primarily for patient care. It does have direct input for clinical research and use in community hospitals and in developing countries for providing quality-controlled cancer data for end-results reporting.

Staging Soft Tissue Sarcoma — AJCC

Soft tissue sarcomas arise in a variety of tissues in all parts of the body — fibrous connective tissue; fat, smooth or striated muscle, vascular tissue, and peripheral neural tissue, as well as from poorly-differentiated mensenchyme.

This GTNM classification applies to all soft tissue sarcomas, except Kaposi's sarcoma, dermatofibrosarcoma, and desmoid type of fibrosarcoma, Grade I. Excluded from the staging system are those sarcomas arising within

Pinedo, H.M., Verweij, J., and H.D. Suit (eds.): Soft Tissue Sarcomas: New Developments in the Multidisciplinary Approach to Treatment. © 1991 Kluwer Academic Publishers, Boston. ISBN: 0-7923-1139-6. All rights reserved.

the confines of the dura mater, including the brain, and sarcomas arising in parenchymatous organs and hollow viscera.

The classification and staging system is based upon analysis of 1,215 cases of soft tissue sarcoma obtained from 13 institutions; cases were collected on the basis of the histology, diagnosis, and type of soft tissue sarcoma and included all age groups [3]. For the most part, recommendations regarding the staging of soft tissue sarcomas in children are the same as the AJCC system for adults.

Histologic Types

The following histopathologic tumor types are those comprising study analysis in the data base and represent the types upon which the staging was determined for the system.

Alveolar soft-part sarcoma
Angiosarcoma
Epithelioid sarcoma
Extraskeletal chondrosarcoma
Extraskeletal osteosarcoma
Fibrosarcoma
Leiomyosarcoma
Liposarcoma
Malignant fibrous histiocytoma
Malignant hemangiopericytoma
Malignant mesenchymoma
Malignant schwannoma
Rhabdomyosarcoma
Synovial sarcoma
Sarcoma, NOS (not otherwise specified)

Classification — GTNM

Histopathologic grade (G):
Malignancy grade is required for staging soft tissue sarcoma. This assessment by a qualified pathologist, made from a representative sampling of the tumor, is the most significant contributing value factor for sarcoma staging, being reflective of potential for recurrence,tumor sensitivity for therapy, and prognosis evaluation. Accordingly, a grade symbol (G) was added to the TNM symbols. Using the accepted criteria of malignancy, the tumor is graded as follows:

GX   grade cannot be assessed
G1   well-differentiated
G2   moderately-well-differentiated
G3   poorly-differentiated; undifferentiated

Extent of primary tumor (T):
  TX primary tumor cannot be assessed
  T0 no evidence of primary tumor
  T1 tumor 5 cm or less in greatest dimension
  T2 tumor more than 5 cm in greatest dimension

Regional lymph node metastasis (N):
  NX regional lymph nodes cannot be assessed
  N0 no regional lymph node metastasis
  N1 regional lymph node metastasis

Distant metastasis (M):
  MX presence of distant metastasis cannot be assessed
  M0 no distant metastasis
  M1 distant metastasis

Stage Grouping

Stage I: A — G1, T1, N0, M0
               well-differentiated tumor, 5 cm or less in greatest
               dimension, no regional lymph nodal or distant metasta-
               sis
               B — G1, T2, N0, M0
               well-differentiated tumor, more than 5 cm in greatest
               dimension, no regional lymph nodal or distant metasta-
               sis
Stage II: A — G2, T1, N0, M0
               moderately-well-differentiated tumor, 5 cm or less in
               greatest dimension, no regional lymph nodal or distant
               metastasis
               B — G2, T2, N0, M0
               moderately-well-differentiated tumor, more than 5 cm
               in greatest dimension, no regional lymph nodal or dis-
               tant metastasis
Stage III: A — G3, T1, N0, M0
               poorly-differentiated or undifferentiated tumor, 5 cm or
               less in greatest dimension, no regional lymph nodal or
               distant metastasis
               B — G3, T2, N0, M0
               poorly-differentiated or undifferentiated tumor, more
               than 5 cm in greatest dimension, no regional lymph
               nodal or distant metastasis
Stage IV: A — any G, any T, N1, M0
               tumor of any differentiation, any size, with regional
               lymph nodal metastasis but without distant metastasis

B — any G, any T, any N, M1
> tumor of any differentiation, any size, with or without regional lymph nodal metastasis, with distant metastasis

An analysis of 702 cases (from the 1215 case data base) with totally complete staging data on each case demonstrated 5-year survival rates of 75% for Stage I, 55% for Stage II, 29% for Stage III, and 7% for Stage IV [3].

Variations of TNM System

There are two other systems in addition to the AJCC/UICC staging.

The Hajdu system has added to the TNM the depth of tumor extension from the surface in its stage determination for surgical evaluation and survival information [4].

The Musculoskeletal Tumor Society (MTS) has further adapted the TNM for tumors of the extremities; as such, it does not employ "N" for assessment of lymph nodal involvement. However, the MTS system is unique in providing for the staging of benign tumors as well as malignant tumors. The MTS symbols designated malignancy grade (G), anatomic site of the tumor (T), and metastasis (M). Malignancy grade has been subdivided into benign (G_0), low grade (G_1), and high grade (G_2). Tumor site is sub-divided into intracapsular (T_0); extracapsular, intracompartmental (T_1); and, extracapsular, extracompartmental (T_2). (See Chapter 4.)

Conclusion

A TNM staging of soft tissue sarcomas provides valued information for the treating physicians in the selection of the therapies for maximization of results for greatest survival. Although primarily designed for patient care, TNM staging provides a specially-valued contribution for clinical research with quality-controlled data for end results reporting.

The research contribution notwithstanding, TNM staging contributes its greatest benefit in sarcoma treatment from its accessibility and ease of application for discovery by primary care and referral physicians in community hospitals and in developing countries. The letter and symbol agreement of the AJCC and UICC on TNM staging, establishing a worldwide agreement on staging cancer, enhances these benefits.

References

1. American Joint Committee on Cancer Manual for staging of Cancer, 3rd edition. Beahrs OH, Henson DE, Hutter RVP, Myers MH (eds). Philadelphia: Lippincott JB, 1988.

2. Hutter RVP: At last — world-wide agreement on the staging of cancer. Presidential Address, 39th Annual Meeting of the Society of Surgical Oncology, London. Arch Surg 122:1235—1239, 1987.
3. Russell WO, Cohen J, Enzinger F, et al.: A clinical and pathological staging system for soft tissue sarcomas. Cancer 40:1562—1570, 1977.
4. Hajdu SI: Differential diagnosis of soft tissue and bone tumors. Philadelphia: Lea and Febiger, 1986.
5. Enneking WF, Spanier SS, Goodman MA: A system for the surgical staging of musculoskeletal sarcoma. Clin Orthop 153:106—120, 1980.
6. Enneking WF: A system of staging musculoskeletal neoplasms. Clin Orthop 204:9—24, 1986.
7. Suit HD, Mankin HJ, Wood WC, Gebhardt MC, Marmon DC, Rosenberg A, Tepper JE, Rosenthal D: Treatment of the patient with stage M_0 sarcoma of soft tissue. J Clin Oncol 6:854—862, 1988.

4. Principles of Surgical Treatment of Soft Tissue Sarcomas

Henry J. Mankin, Dempsey S. Springfield, and Mark C. Gebhardt

Introduction

Soft tissue tumors are uncommon and in fact, by standards of many other afflictions and ills of the species, do not constitute a major health hazard in any country. In the U.S. soft tissue sarcomas comprise less than 1% of all newly diagnosed cancers per year and lag far behind the various epithelial and glandular lesions (compare 143,000 new cases of adenocarcinoma of the breast in the U.S. in 1989 with less than 5,000 soft tissue sarcomas in the same period!).

Despite their infrequency, the tumors of the somatic soft tissues hold a certain fascination for the orthopedist and surgical oncologist, since unlike adenocarcinomas of the breast or squamous cell carcinomas of the lung, which are limited to one anatomical site and have fairly stereotypic clinical presentations, tumors of soft tissue represent a truly remarkable panoply of histologic diagnoses, clinical presentations, and biologic behaviors — so extraordinary in some cases that defining (and naming) the lesion can occupy as much (or more) time as treating it! To illustrate that point, one need only review the listing of tumor types defined in the tables from the various texts [1,2] or elsewhere in this volume (see Chapter 1). As can readily be noted, each of the component elements of the soft somatic tissues has at least one representative, and several have many. To make matters even more complex, some of these are benign, and others malignant. Among the malignant tumors, some are known to be high grade and have a reputation for early metastatic spread, while others are thought to be a lesser threat to the patient. Perhaps the most confounding feature however is that some of the lesions are deceptive — seemingly bland on histologic study, but displaying a remarkably aggressive course — while others appear as high grade lesions, but rarely cause the patient much harm.

In consideration of the principles of surgical management of soft tissue tumors, the subject is as broad as the distribution of the various lesions. There is considerable difference between the management one might propose for a lipoma of the buttock from that for an epithelioid sarcoma of the forearm, while the management of a rhabdomyosarcoma of the thigh would

Pinedo, H.M., Verweij, J., and H.D. Suit (eds.): Soft Tissue Sarcomas: New Developments in the Multidisciplinary Approach to Treatment. © 1991 Kluwer Academic Publishers, Boston. ISBN: 0–7923–1139–6. All rights reserved.

differ from both. Nevertheless, there are some principles that can be enunciated and, if followed, may make the difficult cases a bit easier.

Axioms

If one is to deal with soft tissue tumors in any sort of rational fashion, it is important to remember a few axioms that, although not always valid, represent "road markers" that help guide the way along an often difficult course.
   The axioms include:
1. Soft tissue tumors are often malignant or aggressive (more so than their bony counterparts) and, with rare exception, should be carefully evaluated prior to either surgically excising them or reassuring the patient that they need not worry.
2. Large lesions are more likely to be malignant than are small ones. (This statement implies a "relativity" to the size of the anatomical part in which the lesion is located. Thus, a cherry-sized lesion of the thigh is theoretically less likely to be malignant than the same sized tumor in the palm of the hand.)
3. Superficially placed small lesions are less likely to be malignant (with the exception of the epithelioid sarcoma and dermatofibrosarcoma protuberans). More deeply placed ones should be viewed with greater suspicion.
4. Tumors tend to behave in a fashion reminiscent of the parent tissue (thus displaying an "organoid" tendency), and hence, the liposarcoma is often relatively avascular, while the angiosarcoma is very bloody; the neurofibroma and neurofibrosarcoma run along nerve trunks, and the fibrosarcoma tends to arise from fascial planes. One must be a bit careful in applying this rule to excess, since only rarely does synovial sarcoma arise within a joint!
5. Some tumors can be present for many years and never seem to change (lipomas, fibromas, neurofibromas, etc.), while others can appear suddenly and become enormous in a relatively short period of time (most often the malignant tumors). However, some are deceptive in that they may be present for years without change and then suddenly "take off". Such prolonged histories are common with synovial sarcoma.
6. If the soft tissue tumor has calcification within it, it is most likely to be a hemangioma or an arteriovenous malformation. If a malignant soft tissue tumor is found to have calcifications on x-ray or CT, the synovial sarcoma or liposarcoma are the two most frequent to present in such a way.
7. Malignant fibrous histiocytoma, fibrosarcoma, and synovial sarcoma, more often than not, present in the lower extremity, especially the thigh and pelvis, while the epithelioid and clear cell sarcomas tend to present in the upper extremity. Fibromatosis (desmoid) is most common around the foot and ankle and rarely appears in the hand and wrist; synovial chon-

dromatosis and giant cell tumor of the tendon sheath seem to prefer the hand and far less commonly appear in the foot.

8. Patients with neurofibromatosis are very likely to develop a neurofibrosarcoma, and conversely, anyone who presents with a neurofibrosarcoma should be studied for evidence of underlying von Recklinghausen's disease.

9. Regardless of the pathological designation and tissue of origin of the lesion and indeed independent of anatomical site, the most important determinant of the biological behavior and the ultimate outcome is the histological grade as defined by a pathological examination of the tissue (benign, 1, 2, or 3). So in fact, a grade 3 leiomyosarcoma is more likely to metastasize than a grade 2 liposarcoma, which in turn is more likely to do harm to the patient than a grade 1 synovial sarcoma, which is more of a threat to the patient than a benign fibrous histiocytoma!

Staging Systems

Although staging systems and work-up of the patient are covered in other sections of this treatise, several comments are included here, as planning the surgery is so heavily dependent upon the staging algorithm. The introduction of usable staging systems has been a major advance in the management of patients with sarcoma of soft tissues and makes surgical planning, management, and result analysis much simpler. Defining the extent of disease by a systematic assessment of histological grade (G), local anatomy (T), and presence/absence of nodal (N) or distant metastasis (M) has not only provided clinicians a common language, but offers a powerful tool for the determination of prognosis [7]. The AJC/UICC [8] staging system is preferred by our group, as the T designation is based upon tumor size, and G designation is a three-step function.

The Staging Algorithm

The information required to define the stage of a soft tissue lesion by any system, as cited above, can be obtained by an algorithmic approach to the patient. The essential data are those that define the grade, anatomical extent (and size) of the tumor, and the presence or absence of nodal and/or distant metastases. Numerous protocols have been described [2,3,9,10,11,12,13], but the one that seems to provide the most information for the least effort is the following:

1. History and physical examination with special attention to regional lymph nodes and abdominal masses.
2. Biplanar x-rays of the part.

3. Chest x-ray (PA and right lateral) and computerized tomography (CT) of the chest.
4. CT and/or magnetic resonance imaging (MRI) of the lesional site (the latter study is more likely to provide the critical information [see below]).
5. ^{99M}Tc diphosphonate bone scan if the lesion is located near a bone or if metastases to a bone are suspected.
6. Angiography (not used very frequently today, but may be useful in defining the location of the blood vessels and their encasement by a tumor prior to surgical resection).
7. Staging abdominal CT and laboratory studies (CBC, ESR, liver function studies, bone marrow, etc.) to help rule out abscess, granuloma, metabolic disease, lymphoma, etc.

Magnetic resonance imaging has been one of the most valuable of the newer techniques in the assessment of soft tissue tumors (see Chapter 2). The use of this modality has eliminated in large measure the need for angiography or lymphangiograms and has provided very accurate definitions of the anatomical placement of the tumor, the containment or lack of containment of the tumor in a compartment, volume measurements, and the relationship to adjacent structures. These data have materially aided the surgeon in planning resective surgery. In most instances, the T2-weighted images provide a considerably better definition of the margins and extent of the disease than do T1 or the CT images, both of which are often less distinct [14,15,16,17,18,19].

The data obtained from these studies should provide a "T" (defined by the physical examination, x-ray, bone scan, CT, MRI, and/or angiography) and an "M" (physical examination, CT of the chest, staging abdominal CT, laboratory studies, and bone scan). The "G" can only be determined by histological examination of material obtained by biopsy.

Biopsy of Soft Tissue Sarcomas

The definitive diagnosis for a tumor of the soft tissues is made on the basis of an analysis of a specimen of tissue obtained by biopsy. Although considered by some to be a minor procedure (and by at least one group of respected surgeons to be unnecessary for certain tumors of the soft tissues [13,20]), in the authors' opinion, the biopsy remains a critical and central part of the staging system. It should be carefully planned, reviewed with other members of the staging team, and performed by an experienced and senior individual. One of the most important issues that arises with the biopsy is that all aspects of it must be considered in the light of any potential subsequent surgical procedure (local or wide resection and/or amputation). The biopsy skin incision and soft tissue track must be placed in an anatomical site that can be subsequently resected in continuity with the specimen containing the tumor, regardless of the type of resective surgery or amputation that is ultimately required to obtain local control. Because of the critical nature of these considerations, wherever possible the biopsy should be done at an institution where the subsequent definitive treatment will be performed [21,22].

Most surgical oncologists believe that an *incisional* biopsy (whether by open or needle technique), rather than an *excisional* one, is the appropriate method of dealing with a soft tissue lesion in which the diagnosis is unknown [21,23]. The reasoning behind such an approach is related to the now widely advocated use of adjuvant radiation, which is often best given prior to the definitive surgical resection (see below). A second reason is the potential dangers associated with either surgical undertreatment of a malignant lesion or overtreatment of a benign one. Excessive surgery for a benign or low grade lesion is almost as objectionable as incomplete resection of a malignant one.

Not only then is an incisional biopsy advocated by most surgeons for the diagnosis of soft tissue tumors, but many centers require that the biopsy be performed by an open technique chiefly because initial studies of the tissue now demand a rather large segment of tissue for analysis (often more than one can get with a needle). The purpose of the biopsy is to obtain sufficient tissue not only for histologic diagnosis of the lesion, but also for additional studies that may in fact be equally important in the management of the patient. Most surgeons try to obtain sufficient tissue for culture, histology, histochemistry, immunoperoxidase staining studies for histochemical markers, electron microscopy, flow cytometry, and other studies [24,25, 26,27,28,29].

Perhaps equally concerning is the possibility that the needle biopsy will be taken from a nonrepresentative area of the tumor and thus provide a somewhat happier picture than actually exists. Such a problem is more frequent with bone tumors, especially those arising from cartilage, but occasionally a high grade neurofibrosarcoma or liposarcoma seems to arise from a less malignant (and sometimes benign) underlying pathological state.

Despite these statements, it should be clearly noted that there is a place for a needle biopsy in soft tissue tumor surgery, and a number of centers use that method routinely and almost exclusively. The several techniques available will be described below.

If the surgeon decides that an open biopsy is necessary, the procedure should be carefully planned and reviewed in advance with the pathologist who must deal with the tissue to be obtained. The wound should be small and placed in an anatomical site that can be subsequently resected during the definitive procedure (see above). Transverse incisions in the extremities, although often providing a better cosmetic result, are very difficult to excise in subsequent procedures and make extensile exposure difficult. The transverse biopsy incision in itself is at times an iatrogenic cause for amputation in a patient who might otherwise be treated by a limb-sparing procedure [21,23].

In regard to the deeper tissues, it is considered safest is to go *through* muscle rather than along fascial planes. Muscle that is contaminated by the biopsy can be readily resected with the specimen at the time of definitive surgery. Traversing tissue planes (such as the interosseous membrane separating the anterior from the posterior compartment of the arm), although considerably "neater" and less bloody, contaminate both compartments and may markedly increase the extent of the definitive surgery required to eliminate the neoplasm.

The use of a pneumatic tourniquet is debated by surgical oncologists, and many do not use these devices at the time of either biopsy or definitive resection. The theoretical objection (never proven!) is related to the "damming" effect of the tourniquet. Manipulation of the tumor during the procedure is thought to result in increased shedding of cells that, in theory at least, accumulate in the veins at the tourniquet margin and adhere to one another to form large clumps. At the time of release of the tourniquet, it is postulated that the cell masses enter the venous tree and are widely distributed through the lungs. The masses, if sufficient cells adhere to one another, may be large enough to be trapped in the pulmonary vascular tree and, perhaps more logically, have a greater chance of survival than single cells when implanted in foreign sites. It should be emphasized that this theory, although reasonable, remains unproven, and in fact, the author and his colleagues frequently use a tourniquet to avoid excessive bleeding or to decrease the amount of tissue injury sustained in a deep biopsy.

Regardless of whether or not a tourniquet is used, the surgeon should strive for careful hemostasis and a dry field at the time of closure of the biopsy site. Wound closure should be performed in layers, and many surgeons do not drain the site. If a drain seems appropriate, the drain exit site should be closely adjacent and in a linear alignment to either end of the biopsy incision, since it too will have to be resected with the specimen at the time of definitive surgery. Placing the drain site far from the wound may make it impossible to perform a subsequent resection, since the entire field traversed by the drain must be considered contaminated by tumor cells [21].

Tissue should be sent for a frozen section during the biopsy procedure. Although occasionally this provides a definitive diagnosis, the principal purpose of the frozen section is to be certain that pathological tissue is obtained and that a definitive diagnosis is likely to be made by subsequent study of the material. It is also essential to culture the wound even when the lesion is clearly a neoplasm and neither bacterial or fungal abscess is likely. It should be apparent that if the final diagnosis suggests an inflammatory or infectious lesion, having the cultural data is very helpful and can save the day! Sufficient tissue should also be obtained for histology, histochemistry, immunopathological study of the tissue [25,26,27], flow cytometric analysis for DNA kinetics [28,29], and electron microscopy. All of these studies are now considered important in not only defining the nature of the tumor, but, more importantly, in assigning a grade and predicting the biological behavior.

It is clearly possible to obtain a definitive diagnosis of soft tissue sarcoma (and rule out other processes) by needle biopsy without the difficulties and inconvenience of a surgical procedure or the necessity for other than local anesthesia. Numerous devices are available for such procedures, but the most frequently used is a Tru-cut biopsy needle with which sufficient tissue can be obtained to make not only a histological definition, but other studies as well, especially if several cores are obtained [30]. Planning for this procedure should be similar to the exercise surrounding the open biopsy, in that the needle tract of the biopsy may be seeded with tumor and hence will require resection with the specimen at the time of definitive surgery. The biopsy usually is performed using local anesthesia and does not require hospitalization. Aspiration biopsy with a thin needle provides cells for cytodiagnosis, and some centers have claimed excellent results with this less invasive technique [31,32].

In recent years the radiologists have developed a technique for biopsy during computerized tomography visualization, which materially enhances the success rate of the procedure [33]. A fine needle is used to obtain an aspirate of cells for cytodiagnosis; but a more definitive sample may be obtained using the disposable Tru-cut device described above. Although the amount of tissue obtainable is limited by this technique, it is especially valuable for deeply placed lesions, those adjacent to vital structures, or those in which the biopsy site is likely to bleed excessively.

A final consideration is the performance of the "excisional" biopsy rather than the "incisional" one advocated by those who perform either the conventional or needle biopsies described above. As a general rule, performing an excisional biopsy without a definitive diagnosis introduces two hazards: underestimating the extent of a malignant tumor and hence undertreating it; and overestimating the extent of a benign lesion and thus overtreating it. Many surgeons consider this technique appropriate for very small superficially placed lesions or for tumors that on imaging studies are thought to be clearly benign. Lipomas can often be so strongly suspected on the basis of imaging studies that it seems unnecessary to do an incisional biopsy prior to resection; small lesions in the hand or foot, such as a ganglion or giant cell tumor of the tendon sheath or desmoid tumor, in many experienced surgeon's view, need not be biopsied prior to excision. Although this author does not agree, some surgeons have advocated primary excisional biopsy for lesions that appear to be malignant on imaging studies. The proponents of such a technique [13,20] point out that the staging studies are not only quite accurate in defining the extent and perhaps the nature of the lesion, but are almost equally useful in suggesting the grade of the tumor and hence reducing the potential for error to a very low figure in their hands. The claim is that the surgery without the biopsy reduces the incidence of local recurrence and wound complications.

Management of Soft Tissue Tumors

The systems for the rational management of soft tissue tumors vary rather widely from center to center, depending on the preference of the treatment team, but in any circumstance, they depend at least in part on the grade of the lesion, the anatomical site, and the presence or absence of distant metastases (hence, the need for the staging information). Generally speaking, the treatment is best carried out by a team rather than one or another service or individual, and in our institution, most cases are reviewed at a weekly meeting by members of the Orthopedic Service, the Pathology and Radiology Departments, and the Medical Oncologists and Radiation Therapists. All individuals concerned with the case discuss the management including the staging work-up, the advisability and nature of adjunctive treatment, and the extent of the surgical procedures.

In consideration of management systems, four such programs are currently advocated by one or another of the centers that treat many of these lesions. In addition, however, some centers add chemotherapy either prior to the radiation and/or surgery or after (or both) (see Chapters 7 and 8). The following protocols are available:

1. Surgery alone (either resection or amputation) [6,9,13,20].
2. Wide or marginal surgical excision followed by postoperative radiation therapy to the tumor bed [34].
3. Preoperative radiation therapy to the tumor followed, after an appropriate interval, by marginal or wide excision, and followed at an appropriate interval by a subsequent radiation boost to achieve a tumorocidal dose to the bed [35,36,37].
4. Radiation alone. This program is generally only advised for patients who are too ill to have surgery or who have such wide-spread disease that performing an extensive surgical extirpation or amputation is inappropriate (see Chapter 6).

Before further discussing these approaches to the soft tissue tumors, it seems appropriate to define the types of surgical procedures more clearly, using the classification system devised and reported by Enneking and the Musculoskeletal Tumor Society [7]. The extent and potential disability of the surgical procedures for resection of soft tissue tumors vary according to the anatomical site and the desired amount of normal tissue one wishes to sacrifice (the "margin"). If one considers the procedures generically, both amputations and resections can be described according to the margin obtained, and four types of procedure are described [3,6,10,11,12,38].

The first of these, <u>intralesional</u> occurs, as the name implies, within the tumor and in fact leaves gross tumor behind in the bed. As with all of the other types of procedure as well, either an amputation or resection can be intralesional. Such a procedure is reserved for benign lesions or those that are more aggressive and that, for one reason or another, require a "debulk-

44

ing" procedure. The likelihood of local recurrence following intralesional procedures is high except with some benign tumors.

A second procedure, designed as *marginal*, establishes the resection or amputation margin at the compressed soft tissue capsule that serves as a limiting envelope for the lesion. The "reactive zone" around rapidly growing malignant tumors of soft tissue establishes a plane that allows the tumor to be "shelled out" from the bed, a technically satisfying approach to the problem, which involves little sacrifice of normal tissue and hence the lessened extent of an amputation or disability after resection. The difficulty with this approach however, particularly for high grade tumors or even desmoids (which tend to be highly infiltrative), is that the compressed reactive zone contains not only tongues of tumor tissue, but often satellite daughter nodules. Marginal procedures should be reserved for patients with lesions of low potential for local recurrence or those in which wider procedures are either not possible or potentially severely disabling and for which adjuvant radiation (either pre- or postoperative) will provide the necessary "kill" to the remaining microscopic tumor in order to reduce the rate of local recurrence to an acceptable minimum.

The third type of procedure, termed *wide*, is the standard one used by surgeons for amputation or resection of high grade soft tissue (and bone) tumors. As the term implies a variably sized cuff of normal tissue is left surrounding the lesion and the reactive zone. The resection however remains within the anatomical compartment in which the tumor arises and as such may leave "skip" metastases along vessels or nerve trunks. If done correctly however, the likelihood of a local recurrence after a wide resection (with a centimeter or more of margin) is very low and even further reduced if adjuvant radiation therapy is administered to the bed.

A fourth procedure, known as *radical*, is rarely used today. To achieve radical margins requires removal of the entire compartment in which the tumor arises. Hence, a lesion of the anterior compartment of the thigh treated by a radical procedure would require either a hip disarticulation or a resection of the entire quadriceps muscle mass.

Some general principals regarding the surgery include the obvious fact that it is essential to plan the surgical procedure to include the biopsy wound or tract in the tissue removed during the resection or amputation. This will eliminate the potential for local recurrence as a result of seeding of the biopsy tract with tumor cells. Surgery should be done under tourniquet if there is a threat of major blood loss (see above in the section under "biopsy" for the theoretical objection to the use of a pneumatic tourniquet), and the resection plan based on the imaging studies should be carefully followed to achieve the predetermined margin.

As a general rule, the surgical specimen should be examined in the operating room by the pathologist to be certain that there is no tumor at the margins, and appropriate frozen sections taken at the resection margin of the tumors will provide assurance as to the width of the margin obtained at the surgery. Following the resective or amputative surgery, meticulous care should be taken to achieve hemostasis and a tight closure performed over drains. Both wound drainage and antibiotics should be continued for a reasonable length of time. If preoperative radiation has been performed or if postoperative radiation is contemplated, the sutures should be left in place for longer than usual (sometimes as long as 6 weeks or more). Rehabilitation is facilitated by bracing as necessary and by the prescription of appropriate exercises and mobilization techniques.

In now considering more closely the four protocols introduced above, it should be readily apparent that the management of benign lesions of soft tissue represents little problem [4]. Even large lipomas can be safely resected and indeed "shelled out" without much difficulty. Fibromas, neurolemmomas, myxomas, ganglions, giant cell tumors of the tendon sheath, hemangiomas, arteriovenous malformations, and a number of other benign processes involving the extremities and thorax can be treated effectively by a primary marginal or intralesional surgical procedure, with little threat of complication or recurrence. The lower grade lesions (histological grade 1) still represent a problem, particularly since many surgeons find it difficult to sacrifice vital anatomy for nonmetastasizing tumors even when they behave as aggressively as fibromatosis (desmoid) or dermatofibrosarcoma protuberans do. Although radiation may play a role in the management of such lesions as atypical lipomas and desmoid tumors, the treatment is mostly surgical, and success can almost always be achieved by obtaining a wide or at least a marginal margin.

In terms of malignant lesions arising from the soft tissues, only a few centers advocate the surgical procedure alone, and in past experience, such procedures, unless they were high amputations, had a significant local recurrence rate (over 25%). If radiation is to be used in order to reduce the likelihood of a local failure, it should be emphasized that the treatment plan should adhere to the well-known principles of cancer surgery, and the old dictum still holds that adjuvant radiation or chemotherapy cannot compensate for inadequate or poorly performed surgery.

In our view, the best results will be obtained with a patient with a sarcoma of soft tissues if no prior surgery (even a biopsy) has been done prior to our treatment; the best method of treatment, where possible, is protocol #3 above, which includes preoperative radiation, surgery, and a postoperative boost [35]. The radiation field can be more limited than if one treats postoperatively, and despite a relatively high rate of delayed healing, the ultimate functional outcome is usually quite good.

Such a patient should be staged, biopsied, and then treated with radiation using a diminishing field technique. The radiation is given at 2.0 Gy per day with a 5 day week, and the current protocol suggests that a tumor dose approximating 48 Gy is appropriate. After a 3-week wait, the tumor is resected (preferably with a marginal or wide margin). After wound healing is achieved (hopefully by 2 to 3 weeks), the course of adjuvant radiation is completed by bringing the total dose to 64 to 68 Gy usually by external beam. In selected circumstances, the boost may be given immediately after completion of the resection while the wound is still open (interoperative radiation) or by the use of catheters placed in the wound at the time of closure and into which are implanted a radioactive source (such as iridium). Using these techniques or ones with only slight modifications, our unit has been able to achieve a success rate for local control of the tumor of over 90% [35].

A second somewhat less optimal approach is that defined in protocol #2 above. In this circumstance the lesion is resected, and the radiation given postoperatively. Many of these patients in our center are those treated elsewhere by "shelling out" or marginal surgery. For these patients, our standard protocol is, first, a careful staging; followed by radiation to approximately 48 Gy; and then after a waiting period and restaging, resection of the bed [39]. Overall, this type of surgery is only slightly less successful than the former, but the wound complications are often greater. The radiation field is of necessity considerably broader, and by definition, the patient must undergo two large surgical procedures in a short period of time. The surgical bed is likely to be a poor one based on a diminished vascularity, and wound healing is probably more of a problem in this group than in those patients treated with radiation preoperatively [36].

In terms of avoiding or treating wound complications, it should be clearly evident that either management system defined above introduces some special problems in the surgical therapy of the patient and may introduce a significant potential for poor wound healing. If preoperative radiation is given, the surgery should be delayed at least 2 weeks (perhaps as long as three is even better) following completion of the radiation. Wound treatment during the operative procedure should be appropriately gentle (as in any good surgical procedure, but especially in this setting and in the extremities, since the skin and soft tissues may be less forgiving than in other tissues), and when possible, the wound should be carefully planned to avoid unusual configurations, sharp angulations, or wide separations that can only be closed under tension. If it is possible to save some of the underlying muscle and especially the deep fascia subjacent to the skin, the likelihood of skin slough (a dreaded complication of such a procedure) may be sharply reduced. Wound closure should in general be in layers, with attempts made to pull viable muscle layers over the resection bed.

If at the time of planning the procedure or after resecting the tumor and during the wound closure it is thought that the viability of the skin and subjacent soft tissues is in peril, it is appropriate to plan for some plastic surgical maneuver that may materially improve the viability of the soft tissue cover over the radiated bed and enhance the likelihood of primary healing of the surgical wound. Some of the techniques often utilized include local muscle flaps (gastrocnemius, soleus and rectus flaps for the lower extremity,

47

latissimus dorsi and pectoralis major flaps for the upper). In many of these approaches, the viable and usually nonradiated muscle on a neurovascular pedicle is lifted from its insertion or origin and redirected into the wound site and subsequently covered with a split skin graft [40] or free pedicle flaps, principally using the latissimus dorsi muscle transplanted on a vascular pedicle anastamosed to a local artery and vein [41]. The latter procedure may or may not include a surface layer of skin, but more commonly includes a split skin graft cover. The free flap is the most complex of the skin coverage procedures, takes the longest time (sometimes up to 8 additional hours of surgery), and since it opens up a new operative field, increases at least the theoretical hazard of transplantation of tumor cells. Nevertheless, for some wounds in some anatomical sites, this procedure is of great value in providing skin coverage and inducing rapid functional recovery in a setting that would almost surely have failed to heal if more conventional treatment methods were employed [42].

Regardless of the method utilized to achieve a tight wound closure without tension, it is essential that that the wound site be drained to avoid a fluid collection in a dead space. Radiated wounds or those in patients on prolonged chemotherepeutic regimens often show rather remarkable degrees of sterile serosanginous fluid production, which may persist for days or even weeks following the surgery. The early use of multiple drains to minimize the space in which the fluid is likely to accumulate, as well as a pressure dressing (a Robert Jones cotton-elastic bandage wrap is preferred by the authors), may be helpful in minimizing this complication. The extremity should be put at rest, and although exercises should be started as soon as feasible to avoid stiff joints, too early movement of the wound site may lead to poor healing or wound dehiscence. It is appropriate in some cases to avoid moving the joints through other than a few degrees of motion for as long as 2 or more weeks for some wounds, and the same applies to the elbow or shoulder areas (although the last mentioned is more likely to heal because of the rich vascular supply of the region).

If the remainder of the radiation is to be given to the bed following the surgery or if chemotherapy is to be (re)started, it is wise to wait at least 2 weeks following extensive surgical extirpation of especially the large lesions. Sutures should remain in place until the treatment is over (sometimes as long as 6 or more weeks), and careful attention paid to signs of wound breakdown, infection, or fluid accumulation. Ultrasound or CT are very helpful in diagnosing the presence of a fluid accumulation, and at times repeated aspirations, firm dressings, and rest to the part can eliminate this complication.

In consideration of wound healing in patients with soft tissue tumors with or without pre- or postoperative adjuvant radiation and chemotherapy, it is reasonable to remember that the same risk factors that make wound healing problematical in any site may exist in these patients and, because of the nature of the surgery and the use of the adjuvants, remarkably compound the problem. Specifically, the elderly patient with poor peripheral blood supply or the diabetic patient both run a greater risk of wound breakdown, infection, or delayed healing. Patients who are obese have an added risk of difficulties with wound closure and skin necrosis, and those who have been on medications, such as corticosteroids or chemotherepeutic agents, or have some form of connective tissue disorder may in fact present major problems as a result of poor wound healing. It is sometimes advisable to suggest to such patients that an amputation may be a more conservative approach to the problem and will markedly improve the likelihood of rapid return to function than the more complex (and much more likely to be complicated) limb-sparing procedure.

Surgical Management of Metastases

In any series of patients with high grade soft tissue sarcomas, the percentage that develop pulmonary metastases vary from 25 to 40%, and as has been emphasized in recent reports, the larger the primary lesion, the more likely is a metastasis to occur. The estimate in our center for patients with tumors over 15 cm in the longest diameter is that 80% will either present with or develop metastases within 2 years [35].

Furthermore, it is apparent that nodal metastases are not uncommon in tumors of the somatic soft tissues, with the synovial, epitheliod, and clear cell sarcomas leading the list (estimated at up to 15% of the cases) [5,43]. Some of the tumors have a tendency for bony metastasis (in some cases without discernible lesions in the lung), and recent evidence has suggested that about 50% of liposarcomas that metastasize do so to bones and viscera without creating deposits in the lungs [44]. As discussed in Chapter 8 and briefly described below, the view that chemotherapy has an effect on suppressing or eliminating the threat of pulmonary metastases is not well supported by studies (see Chapter 8), and all of this suggests that currently the surgeon, radiation therapist, and oncologist can treat the local lesion often quite effectively, but can only wait to see if the patients will develop metastases and, if they do, hope that their placement and number are such that resection is possible [12,44,45].

Radiation and/or surgical resection of nodal metastases is often successful in reducing this problem. The principle difficulties lie not with the nodes resected, but with the ones beyond the resected (and/or radiated) site and further up the chain. All patients with nodal disease must have a careful CT and/or MRI to ascertain the presence or absence of abnormal nodes in the abdomen or thorax, and they should be carefully followed after resective surgery [43].

Resection of pulmonary nodules occurring in patients with high grade soft tissue sarcomas is sometimes as rewarding as reported for other lesions, such as osteosarcomas, where the 5-year remission rate is considered by some to be as high as 30% [46]. It should be noted however that the chemotherapy of osteosarcoma has been shown to be effective and that treatment both before and after pulmonary resection for metastases is likely to have a profound effect on the outcome. In general, most surgeons feel that the appropriate approach to these problems is chemotherapy and resection (particularly if the number or location of the tumors does not make the procedure untenable) [45,47-49]. A followup period of continued chemotherapy is mandatory, and the patient should be carefully watched at essentially 2-month intervals for evidence of recurrence.

Conclusions

It should be evident that the management of benign tumors of the somatic soft tissues is not a great challenge to the experienced surgeon, and the surgical treatment of hemangiomas, arteriovenous malformations, myxomas, ganglions, giant cell tumors of the tendon sheath, neurolemmomas, lipomas, etc. can be done with little resultant deficit or threat of recurrence. Of considerably greater challenge are the lesions of low or high grade malignancy in which meticulous staging must be carried out, a biopsy performed with strict adherence to a set of rules, and a treatment protocol introduced that is not only multidisciplinary, but requires a form of surgical procedure that the average orthopedist or general surgeon is not always prepared to do. Management of such lesions is complex and, if the rules defined above are not closely adhered to, can lead to recurrent tumor, serious wound complications, functional impairment, and the threat of distant nodal and pulmonary metastases. As potentially grim as are these threats of failure, in sharp contrast are the sweet rewards of successful management that provides a suffering patient with a long-standing remission or cure and a functional extremity.

References

1. Enzinger F, Weiss S: Soft tissue tumors, 2nd edition. St. Louis: CV Mosby, 1988.
2. Hajdu SI: Pathology of soft tissue tumors. Philadelphia: Lea and Febiger, 1979.
3. Creighton JJ, Jr, Peimer CA, Mindell ER, Boone DC, Karakousis CP, Douglass HO: Primary malignant tumors of the upper extremity: Retrospective analysis of one hundred twenty six cases. J Hand Surg [Am] 10:805—814, 1985.
4. Shenaq SM: Benign skin and soft tissue tumors of the hand. Clin Plast Surg 14:403—412, 1987.
5. Hoopes JE, Graham WP, III, Shack RB: Epithelioid sarcoma of the upper extremity. Plast Reconstr Surg 75:810—815, 1985.
6. Rydholm A: Management of patients with soft-tissue tumors. Acta Orthop Scand 54:1—77, 1983.
7. Enneking WF, Spanier SS, Goodman MA: Current concepts review: The surgical staging of musculoskeletal sarcoma. J Bone Joint Surg 62A:1027—1030, 1980.

8. American Joint Committee on Cancer: Manual for staging of cancer, 3rd edition. Philadelphia: JB Lippincott, 1988.
9. Rydholm A, Alvegard T, Berg NO, Dawiskiba Z, Egund N, Idvall I, Pettersson H, Rooser B, Willen H, Akerman M: Preoperative diagnosis of soft tissue tumours. Int Orthop 12:109—114, 1988.
10. Eilber FR: Soft tissue sarcomas of the extremity. Curr Probl Cancer 8:3—41, 1984.
11. Lawrence W, Jr: Concepts in limb-sparing treatment of adult soft tissue sarcomas. Semin Surg Oncol 4:73—77, 1988.
12. Bell RS, O'Sullivan B, Liu FF, Powell J, Langer F, Fornasier VL, Cummings B, Miceli PN, Hawkins N, Quirt I, et al.: The surgical margin in soft tissue sarcoma. J Bone Joint Surg 71A:370—375, 1989.
13. Berlin O, Markhede G, Stener AR, Rooser B, Persson, BM: Deep seated soft tissue sarcomas in the extremities: Long-term results of primary surgical treatment based on clinical diagnosis or aspiration cytology. In: Limb salvage musculoskeletal oncology. Enneking WF (ed). New York: Churchill Livingstone, pp 531—539, 1987.
14. Pettersson H, Eliasson J, Egund N, Rooser B, Willen H, Rydholm A, Berg NO, Holtas S: Gadolinium DTPA enhancement of soft tissue tumors in magnetic resonance imaging: Preliminary clinical experience in five patients. Skeletal Radiol 17:319—323, 1988.
15. Kalmar JA, Eick JJ, Merritt CR, Shuler SE, Miller KD, McFarland GB, Jones JJ: A review of applications of MRI in soft tissue and bone tumors. Orthopedics 11:417—25, 1988.
16. Kilcoyne RF, Richardson ML, Porter BA, Olson DO, Greenlee TK, Lanzer W: Magnetic resonance imaging of soft tissue masses. Clin Orthop 228:13—19, 1988.
17. Chang AE, Matory YL, Dwyer AJ, Hill SC, Girton ME, Steinberg SM, Knop RH, Frank JA, Hyams D, Doppman JL, et al.: Magnetic resonance imaging versus computed tomography in the evaluation of soft tissue tumors of the extremities. Ann Surg 205:340—348, 1987.
18. Aisen AM, Martel W, Braunstein EM, McMillin KI, Phillips WA, Kling TF: MRI and CT evaluation of primary bone and soft tissue tumors. AJR 146:749—756, 1986.
19. Kransdorf MJ, Jelinek JS, Moser RP, Jr, Utz JA, Brower AC, Hudson TM, Berrey BH: Soft tissue masses: Diagnosis using MR imaging. AJR 153:541—547, 1989.
20. Rydholm A, Rooser B, Persson BM: Primary myectomy for sarcoma. J Bone Joint Surg 68A:586—589, 1986.
21. Mankin HJ, Lange TA, Spanier SS: The hazards of biopsy in patients with malignant primary bone and soft-tissue tumors. J Bone Joint Surg 64A:1121—1127, 1982.
22. Rydholm A, Berg NO, Persson BM, Akerman M: Treatment of soft-tissue sarcoma should be centralised. Acta Orthop Scand 54:333—339, 1983.
23. Simon MA: Biopsy of musculoskeletal tumors. J Bone Joint Surg 64A:1253—1257, 1982.
24. Leyvraz S, Costa J: Histological diagnosis and grading of soft tissue sarcomas. Semin Surg Oncol 4:3—6, 1988.
25. duBolay CE: Immunohistochemistry of soft tissue tumours: A review. J Pathol 146:77—94, 1985.
26. Baumal R, Kahn HJ, Bailey D, Phillips MJ, Hanna W: The value of immunohistochemistry in increasing diagnostic precision of undifferentiated tumours by the surgical pathologist. Histochem J 16:1061—1070, 1984.
27. Roholl PJ, DeJong AS, Ramaekers FC: Application of markers in the diagnosis of soft tissue tumours. Histopathology 9:1019—1035.
28. Kreicbergs A, Tibukait B, Willems J, Bauer HCF: Flow DNA analysis of soft tissue tumors. Cancer 59:128—133, 1987.
29. Matsuno T, Gebhardt MC, Schiller AL, Rosenberg AE, Mankin HJ: The use of flow cytometry as a diagnostic aid in the management of soft-tissue tumors. J Bone Joint Surg 70A:751—759.
30. Kissin MW, Fisher C, Carter RL, Horton LW, Westbury G: Value of Tru-cut biopsy in the diagnosis of soft tissue tumours. Br J Surg 73:742—746, 1986.

51

31. Akerman M, Rydholm A: Aspiration cytology of lipomatous tumors: A 10 year experience at an orthopedic oncology center. Diagn Cytopathol 3:295—302, 1987.

32. Miralles TG, Gosalbez F, Menendez P, Astudillo A, Torre C, Buesa J: Fine needle aspiration cytology of soft tissue lesions. Acta Cytol 30:671—678, 1986.

33. Bland KI, McCoy DM, Kinard RE, Copeland EM, , III: Application of magnetic resonance imaging and computerized tomography as an adjunct to the surgical management of soft tissue sarcomas. Ann Surg 205:473—481, 1987.

34. Lindberg RD, Martin RG, Romsdahl MM, Barkley HT: Conservative surgery and post-operative radiotherapy in 300 adults with soft tissue sarcomas. Cancer 47:2391—2397, 1981.

35. Suit HD, Mankin HJ, Wood WC, Gebhardt MC, Harmon DC, Rosenberg A, Tepper JE, Rosenthal D: Treatment of the patient with stage M_0 soft tissue sarcoma. J Clin Oncol 6:854—862, 1988.

36. Mansson E, Willems J, Aparisi T, Jakobsson P, Nilsonne U, Ringborg U: Preoperative radiation therapy of high malignancy grade soft tissue sarcoma. A preliminary investigation. Acta Radiol 22:461—464, 1983.

37. Barkley HT, Martin RG, Romsdahl MM, Lindberg R, Zagard GK: Treatment of soft tissue sarcomas by preoperative irradiation and conservative surgical resection. Int J Rad Oncol Biol Phys 14:693—699, 1988.

38. Rydholm A, Rooser B: Surgical margins for soft-tissue sarcoma. J Bone Joint Surg 69A:1074—1078, 1987.

39. Giuliano AE, Eilber FR: The rationale for planned reoperation after unplanned total excision of soft-tissue sarcomas. J Clin Oncol 3:1344—1348, 1985.

40. Ersek RA, Abell JM, Jr, Calhoon JH: The island pedicle rotation advancement gastro-cnemius musculocutaneous flap for complete coverage of the popliteal fossa. Ann Plast Surg 12:533—536, 1984.

41. Elliott LF, Raffel B, Wade J: Segmental latissimus dorsi free flap: Clinical applications. Ann Plast Surg 23:231—238, 1989.

42. Wexler AM, Eilber FR, Miller TA: Therepeutic and functional results of limb salvage to treat sarcomas of the forearm and hand. J Hand Surg 13:292—296, 1988.

43. Cheng E, Springfield DS, Gebhardt MC: Patterns of metastasis of liposarcoma. Submitted for publication.

44. Ruka W, Emrich LJ, Driscoll DL, Karakousis CP: Prognostic significance of lymph node metastasis and bone, major vessel, or nerve involvement in adults with high-grade soft tissue sarcomas. Cancer 62:999—1006, 1988.

45. Huth JF, Eilber FR: Patterns of metastatic spread following resection of extremity soft-tissue sarcomas and strategies for treatment. Semin Surg Oncol 4:20—26, 1988.

46. Mountain CF, McMurtrey MJ, Hermes KE: Surgery for pulmonary metastasis: A 20-year experience. Ann Thorac Surg 38:323—330, 1984.

47. Jablons D, Steinberg SM, Roth J, Pittaluga S, Rosenberg SA, Pass HI: Metastasectomy for soft tissue sarcoma. Further evidence for efficacy and prognostic indicators. J Thorac Cardiovasc Surg 97:695—705, 1989.

48. Li GH, Li JQ, Cai YH, Huang M: Surgical management of soft tissue sarcomas with an analysis of 313 cases. Semin Surg Oncol 4:82—85, 1988.

49. Rizzoni WE, Pass HI, Wesley MN, Rosenberg SA, Roth JA: Resection of recurrent pulmonary metastases in patients with soft-tissue sarcomas. Arch Surg 121:1248—1252, 1986.

5. Psychological Outcomes in Survivors of Extremity Sarcomas Following Amputation or Limb-Sparing Surgery

William W. Weddington

Introduction

Remarkable progress has occurred regarding surgical techniques and the use of radiation therapy or chemotherapy for the treatment of extremity sarcomas [1-3]. Most patients with extremity sarcomas now have a treatment option of limb-salvage procedures in addition to amputation. Indeed, tumor resection combined with chemotherapy or irradiation have become the treatment of choice for most extremity soft tissue sarcomas [4]. However, patients undergoing limb-salvage surgery require longer periods of anesthesia, several operations, longer hospitalizations, and, consequently, a greater incidence of complications [5]. Yet limb-salvage surgery is increasingly being advocated by surgeons [4], and patients are choosing limb-salvage procedures, perhaps due to a presumption that limb salvage offers preferred outcomes regarding functioning and psychological reactions [6]. Implicit in the endorsement of limb-salvage surgery are presumed psychological advantages of limb-salvage surgery, coupled with an assumption that there are adverse psychological consequences to limb amputation.

Psychosocial Outcomes of Amputation vs. Limb-Salvage Surgery

Surprisingly, there is little information in the medical literature regarding psychological adjustment to surgical interventions by patients with extremity sarcomas. However, several reports exist regarding the psychosocial aspects of limb amputation for cancer.

Boyle and co-workers [7] interviewed 27 adolescents with lower limb amputations secondary to cancer and compared them to data obtained from eight patients with amputations due to trauma at similar ages. Time periods between surgery and interviews ranged from 3 months to 17 years (mean, 7.2 years) for cancer patients and 1 to 7 years (mean, 3.4 years) for traumatic amputees. Among cancer patients, mobility-related activities and social matters, including relations with peers and the opposite sex as well as self-consciousness, were of foremost concern. All cancer survivors who were

Pinedo, H.M., Verweij, J., and H.D. Suit (eds.): Soft Tissue Sarcomas: New Developments in the Multidisciplinary Approach to Treatment. © *1991 Kluwer Academic Publishers, Boston. ISBN: 0–7923–1139–6. All rights reserved.*

amputees considered themselves functionally independent, and 67% had little or no concern for their futures. Although experiences with cancer and amputations significantly impacted patients' lives, a vast majority of patients had a positive view of life, and 85% were determined to have adjusted adequately. The investigators concluded that patients who had undergone amputations due to malignancy differed from traumatic amputees in their adjustment to amputation, with cancer patients showing, in many instances, evidence of better adaptation to disability. However, individuals who underwent amputation for cancer were probably a different group premorbidly than were the trauma patients; thus, comparisons between the two groups are limited.

Tebbi and Mallon [8] examined educational, vocational, and psychosocial states of 20 long-term extremity sarcoma survivors who had undergone amputations during adolescence or early adulthood. When interviewed, all patients had survived for at least 5 years (range 5 to 19 years), were disease free, and were not receiving cancer-related therapy. Eighty-five percent worked at least part time, 85% were either married or dating a steady partner, and nearly 50% had at least some college education. The investigators concluded that the majority of examined patients had adjusted well to their disabilities and led full and functional lives.

Other investigators have examined cancer amputees as part of retrospective analyses of survivors of childhood cancer. O'Malley and associates [9] examined 114 survivors who were diagnosed with cancer when they were younger than 18 years, had a diagnosis of cancer 5 years or longer, were disease free at the time of the interview, and had not received treatment for at least 1 year. Sixteen patients had bone tumors. The researchers determined that the degree of physical impairment secondary to cancer treatment was not significantly related to current psychological adjustments. Patients who adjusted well did so regardless of the degree of physical impairment or insult. In fact, physical impairment was not a variable that distinguished adjusted from maladjusted survivors. Fifty-nine percent of the patients reported mild psychiatric symptoms. Twelve percent were rated as markedly or severely impaired.

Li and Stone [10] evaluated 142 patients who were disease free for at least 5 years after a diagnosis of cancer was made before the age of 18 years. Twenty-eight patients in this series had bone cancer, ten were amputees, and 12 had hypoplastic, weakened, or deformed bones. Sixty-one percent of the patients had attended college. Fifty-three percent were married. Disabling psychological illness attributable to cancer in childhood was uncommon. Moreover, the development of emotional disorders was not clearly related to the presence of severe physical handicaps.

Finally, in another series, Holmes and Holmes [11] examined 124 10-year survivors of childhood cancer. Nineteen of these patients had sarcomas. Ninety survivors reported that the childhood diagnosis of cancer and subsequent treatments had little overall lasting effect on their present lives.

Indeed, there was no significant variance in educational accomplishments and marital experiences with the population at large.

To date there exist only three studies that compare psychological reactions of patients with extremity sarcomas who underwent amputation or limb salvage. Kagan [6], in a descriptive paper regarding adolescent patients' reactions to surgery for extremity osteosarcomas, observed that the emotional rehabilitation of patients undergoing limb-salvage procedures was more difficult compared to that of patients who underwent amputation. Amputees were physically mobile and able to return home after a brief period of time in the hospital compared to limb-salvaged patients. She noted that adolescents who underwent limb-salvage surgery focused their emotional and physical efforts into saving their extremities. On the other hand, amputees, following a brief mourning period subsequent to the loss of their limbs, appeared to adapt to subsequent treatment more easily.

The other two studies compared psychological and social functioning outcomes between adults undergoing amputation or limb-salvage procedures. In the first study, Sugarbaker and colleagues [6] examined 26 young and middle-aged adults with soft tissue sarcomas 1 to 3 years after they underwent amputation plus chemotherapy or limb-sparing surgery and radiation therapy plus chemotherapy. The patients participated in a randomly assigned, controlled clinical trial of treatment for extremity soft tissue sarcomas. After completion of treatment, when patients' physical status had stabilized, the investigators examined adjustment to illness, illness impact, functioning activities of daily living, and an economic assessment. They determined that there were minimal differences between the two groups regarding psychosocial and physical functioning as well as economic costs. Indeed, there was an observable trend toward better performance by amputees as compared to those patients who underwent limb salvage.

At the beginning of the study, the investigators' bias was that the trauma and disability of a major amputation far outweighed the objectionable effects of limb-sparing surgery plus high-dose radiation therapy. Surprised by their findings and concerned by issues regarding the sensitivity and specificy of their psychometric procedures, the researchers developed their own clinical assessments for patients with lower extremity sarcomas. They administered a series of questionnaires that were completed by 23 patients who were still enrolled in the protocol and who had finished chemotherapy, were free of recurrent disease, and had agreed to an evaluation. There were no differences between the group of amputees and limb-salvaged patients regarding pain, mobility, and treatment trauma. However, sexual functioning was more impaired in the limb-spared group as compared to amputees, perhaps as a physiological side effect of radiation therapy.

Finally, in the other study regarding psychological outcomes of extremity sarcoma survivors undergoing amputation or limb-sparing surgery, our group [5] evaluated amputees and patients with salvaged limbs 1 to 5 years after surgery for extremity sarcomas. The patients were being treated by a university-based orthopedic surgeon who specialized in surgical oncology. Over a 5-year period (1978—1982), he had operated on 69 patients aged 14 years or older with extremity sarcomas. Decisions regarding amputation or limb salvage had been reached by a collaborative decision-making process between the surgeon and his patients. However, the surgeon's activity was determined by the grade, location, or extent of the tumor. Thus, patients in the sample were not randomly assigned to treatment.

Of 49 surviving patients who were eligible for an evaluation, we were able to interview 33 patients — 14 amputees and 19 survivors with salvaged limbs. The patients had a variety of soft tissue and bone sarcomas. We administered a cognitive screening examination, a self-administered symptom inventory to examine psychological stress over the prior week, instruments to measure depression and other mood states, and the Karnofsky Performance Scale [13], which assesses the current physical performance and activity states of cancer patients. In addition, we administered a semi-structured psychiatric interview to determine the incidence of past and present psychiatric disorders [14]. The patients had a variety of soft tissue and bone sarcomas. There were no statistically significant differences between the 33 interviewed and the 36 noninterviewed patients with respect to age at surgery, social class, gender, and involved extremities. Nonsurvivors had more chemotherapy, amputations, and a higher incidence of osteosarcoma. The patients had a variety of soft tissue and bone sarcomas.

We found no significant differences between amputees and limb-salvaged patients regarding age, gender, marital status, surgically involved extremity, chemotherapy status, and social class at the time of the interviews. There were no significant differences between the groups in scores of cognitive capacity, symptoms, mood, body image changes, global physical functioning, global adjustment to illness and surgery, and lifetime prevalence of psychiatric disorders before or after surgery. Affective disorders and alcoholism were the most frequently reported lifetime psychiatric disorders. Most patients reported only mild psychological symptoms, and 55% demonstrated good to excellent adjustment to their cancer diseases and surgeries.

In summary, neither Sugarbaker et al. [6] nor members of our group [5] found significant differences in measures of psychological outcomes for patients with extremity sarcomas who underwent limb salvage procedures compared to those who underwent amputation.

Each of the studies described above was limited by sample size; selection bias; study design; sensitivity and specificity of the psychometric instruments, many of which were designed to evaluate psychiatric patients and not medically ill ones; and lack of repeated longitudinal measurements. Thus, there exist definite limitations to generalizing results of these studies to other populations. It is interesting to note that differences have not been found in psychological and social functioning between groups of patients with extremity sarcomas who underwent either amputation or limb-salvage surgery. However, Kagan's [12] work suggests that patients undergoing limb-salvage procedures may experience more acute and short-term adjustment problems than do amputees.

Why No Significant Differences in Psychosocial Outcomes?

Why are the results of these studies surprising? De Haes and van Knippenberg [15] have pointed out that it is commonly assumed that cancer and cancer treatments have a severe, negative impact on the quality of life (QL) of affected patients. However, although significant differences have been found between cancer patients and noncancer patients with respect to some aspects of life, no differences have been found with respect to most QL indicators. They note the extraordinary findings that comparisons between cancer patients and noncancer groups do not support the assumption that the QL of cancer patients in general is poorer than the QL of other groups. In reviewing the literature on the QL of cancer patients, they point out that it has been generally accepted on the basis of intuition and empirical study that cancer and cancer treatments cause a major disruption of life emotionally, socially, and physically. The researchers suggest that psychological mechanisms may, in part, account for the absence of self-reported differences between cancer patients and noncancer populations and may therefore explain the established inconsistencies.

De Haes and van Knippenberg [15] also have pointed out that cancer and cancer treatments influence the QL less than is generally expected. Given that cancer and cancer treatments are disruptive to lives of cancer patients and that reports by patients regarding their QL are subjective, psychological mechanisms must play a part. It is important to note that no systematic studies have been performed to investigate the impact of cancer or cancer treatment on different areas of QL or on overall QL (15).

Patients with cancer appear to "adapt" or "compensate" or "accommodate" psychologically to their diseases, treatments, and possible disabilities. In a study that compared self-reported depressive symptoms in 99 hospitalized patients with advanced cancer, 66 next of kin, and 99 physically healthy persons who were hospitalized because of attempted suicide, Plumb and Holland [16] reported that cancer patients and the next of kin were indistinguishable in psychological or nonsomatic depressive symptoms. Both groups scored lower than the suicide attempters. The researchers noted that the self-esteem of the typical advanced cancer patient and his next of kin was relatively intact. Patients with cancer may be angry at their situation, but they are not angry with themselves. The investigators point out that psychiatric consultation is warranted for patients who demonstrate marked guilt, loss of self-respect, and feelings of worthlessness. They conclude that suppression or repression (unconscious denial) of negative feelings about the future is an important way of coping for cancer patients.

Adaptation, denial, or coping by a patient with cancer may be unappreciated by an observer, care giver, or family member. Indeed, a patient's adaptation may be asynchronous with adaptation to his/her illness by others. Support for the process of adaptation and the proposed phenomenon of asynchronous adaptation is offered by results of a study conducted by Daiter and colleagues [17]. The investigators examined 32 young adult leukemia and lymphoma patients who were newly diagnosed and beginning treatments. Also, the researchers interviewed and evaluated 28 significant peers and family members of the cancer patients. They determined that stress levels were elevated in the group of leukemia and lymphoma patients and that evidence for areas of personal growth were observable. Not surprisingly, stress levels were significantly lower for patients with a more favorable, rather than a less favorable, prognosis. However, patients with a more favorable prognosis were significantly less likely than less favorable prognosis patients to exhibit personal growth or maturation as a result of the illness experience. In contrast, despite elevated stress levels, close social supports of patients with these cancers showed little evidence of similar personal growth.

De Haes and van Knippenberg [15] have reviewed various theoretical explanations for the relatively high QL of cancer patients as well as the patients' ability to adapt. One possible explanation was derived from Helson's adaptation level theory [18]. According to this theory, the adaptation level of a person at any given instant is a weighted geometric mean of all stimuli, past and present, and their effect on the attribute being judged. Thus, the adaptation level will be constantly changing as new experiences are processed. An individual's norms are continually modified by external circumstances. Over the course of their illness, cancer patients change the meaning of different events in their lives to accommodate stressful changes. Worden and Sobel [18] have pointed out in their study of 163 newly diagnosed cancer patients that patients' psychosocial adaptation to cancer was related to their ego strength. They were able to measure adaptation, which was not uniform among the study participants.

Other theories also refer to a continuing adjustment of norms by cancer persons, depending on their life experiences. As a reaction to the stresses of diagnosis and treatment, patients with cancer may come to reappraise various aspects of their lives, such as interpersonal relationships or religious convictions, in such a way that these factors become more meaningful and thus compensate for an increased negative sense of compromised health status [20-24].

Ironically, the attribute of "adaptation" by patients with cancer may affect studies of long-term QL outcomes to cancer and cancer treatments such that no differences in outcomes are noted even between markedly different treatments, such as amputation or limb-salvage surgery, or between cancer patients and noncancer groups. After a diagnosis of cancer and

58

treatments, the score on a given scale may have a different meaning for a cancer patient as compared to his/her precancer or pretreatment perspective or prior pattern of scoring by virtue of his/her experiences with a disease and treatment [14].

Need for Further Research

In addition to more long-term outcome studies of psychosocial or QL changes in cancer patients, there is a need for researchers to focus on repeated measures of short-term psychosocial outcomes following treatment for cancer, in order that we may better understand the phenomenon of psychological adaptation as well as the course of psychosocial changes concurrent with and consequent to diagnosis and treatment. Moreover, if one wishes to examine more thoroughly QL issues in cancer patients in order to compare the impact of treatments on QL, such short-term psychosocial and functioning outcome studies may be more appropriate to tease out differences among treatment outcomes. In addition, there is a need for clearer operational definitions regarding QL, additional studies with larger numbers of patients, and further development of assessment scales to measure the psychological, sexual, and vocational aspects of adjustment to cancer and cancer treatments [25].

Conclusion

There exist several studies of long-term psychosocial and QL outcomes of survivors of extremity sarcomas, including two comparison studies between patients who received amputation or limb-salvage procedures. These studies have revealed that, despite patients with cancer having to experience diseases and treatments that are disruptive to their lives, most patients adapt and report psychosocial and QL outcomes similar to noncancer groups. Psychiatric consultation may be warranted for patients who demonstrate marked guilt, loss of self-respect, or feelings of worthlessness, because these feelings are atypical of the coping process and may indicate clinical depression.

With respect to limb-salvage procedures compared to amputation for extremity sarcomas, a psychological-outcome advantage of limb-salvage surgery has yet to be demonstrated. The absence of differences may occur, in part, because as yet poorly understood psychological adaptive mechanisms are operational. There is a need for further research regarding psychological phenomena of "adaptation" as well as studies of short-term psychosocial and QL outcomes concurrent with and subsequent to various treatment interventions.

References

1. Rosenberg SA, Tepper J, Glatstein E, Costa J, Baker A, Brennan M, Demoss EV, Seipp C, Sindelair WF, Sugarbaker P, Wesley R: The treatment of soft-tissue sarcomas of the extremities. Ann Surg 3:305—315, 1982.
2. Consensus Development Conference on Limb-Sparing Treatment of Adult Soft-Tissue and Osteosarcomas: Limb sparing treatment of adult soft-tissue sarcomas and osteosarcomas. JAMA 254:1791—1796, 1985.
3. Karakonsis CP, Emrich LJ, Krishnamsetty RM: Feasibility of limb salvage and survival in soft tissue sarcomas. Cancer 57:484—491, 1986.
4. Bolton JS, Vauthey JN, Farr GH, Sauter EI, Bowen JC, Kline DG: Is limb-sparing surgery applicable to neurogenic sarcomas of the extremities? Arch Surg 124:118—121, 1989.
5. Weddington WW, Segraves KB, Simon MA: Psychological outcome of extremity sarcoma survivors undergoing amputation or limb salvage. J Clin Oncol 3:1393—1399, 1985.
6. Sugarbaker PH, Barofsky I, Rosenberg SA, Gianola FJ: Quality of life assessment of patients in extremity sarcoma clinical trials. Surgery 91:17—23, 1982.
7. Boyle M, Tebbi CK, Mindell ER, Mettlin CJ: Adolescent adjustment to amputation. Med Pediatr Oncol 10:301—312, 1982.
8. Tebbi CK, Mallon JC: Long-term psychosocial outcome among cancer amputees in adolescence and early adulthood. J Psychosoc Oncol 5:69—82, 1987.
9. O'Malley JE, Koocher G, Foster D: Psychiatric sequelae of surviving childhood cancer. Am J Orthopsychiatry 49:608—616, 1979.
10. Li FP, Stone R: Survivors of cancer in childhood. Ann Intern Med 84:551—553, 1976.
11. Holmes HA, Holmes FF: After ten years, what are the handicaps and life-styles of children treated for cancer? Clin Pediatr 14:819—823, 1975.
12. Kagan LB: Use of denial in adolescents with bone cancer. Health Soc Work 1:71—87, 1976.
13. Karnofsky DA, Burchenal JH: Clinical evaluation of chemotherapeutic agents in cancer. In Evaluation of chemotherapeutic agents. MacLeod CM (ed). New York: Columbia University, pp 33—38, 1949.
14. Weddington WW, Segraves KB, Simon MA: Current and lifetime incidence of psychiatric disorders among a group of extremity sarcoma survivors. J Psychosom Res 30:121—125, 1986.
15. de Haes JCJM, van Knippenberg FCE: The quality of life of cancer patients: A review of the literature. Soc Sci Med 20:809—817, 1985.
16. Plumb MM, Holland J: Comparative studies of psychological functioning in patients with advanced cancer. I. Self-reported depressive symptoms. Psychosom Med 39:264—276, 1977.
17. Daiter S, Larson RA, Weddington WW, Ultmann JE: Psychosocial symptomatology, personal growth, and development among young adult patients following the diagnosis of leukemia or lymphoma. J Clin Oncol 6:613—617, 1988.
18. Helson H, Bevan W: Contemporary approaches to psychology. Princeton, NJ: Van Nostrand, 1967.
19. Worden JW, Sobel HJ: Ego strength and psychosocial adaptation to cancer. Psychosom Med 40:585—592, 1978.
20. Bradburn NM: The structure of psychological well-being. Chicago: Aldine, 1969.
21. Andrews FM, Withey SB: Social indicators of well-being. New York: Plenum Press, 1976.
22. Campbell A, Converse PE, Roders WL: The quality of American life. New York: Sage, 1976.
23. Andrews FM, McKennel AC: Measures of self-reported well-being: Their affective, cognitive and other components. Soc Ind Res 8:127—155, 1980.
24. Meyerowitz BE, Watkins IK, Sparks FC: Quality of life for breast cancer patients receiving adjuvant chemotherapy. Am J Nurs 2:232—235, 1983.
25. Goldberg RT: New trends in the rehabilitation of lower extremity amputees. Rehab Lit 45:2—11, 1984.

6. Radiation Therapy of Sarcomas of the Soft Tissues

Herman D. Suit and Christopher G. Willett

Successful treatment of the patient with sarcoma of soft tissue (STS) means eradication of local, regional, and distant disease, with minimal treatment related morbidity. At present, the potential for such success is limited to those patients who do not have evident metastatic tumors at the time of the diagnosis of the primary tumor. The major exception to this statement is rhabdomyosarcoma in pediatric patients. The American College of Surgeons survey [1] of 5,812 patients treated in U.S. hospitals with A.C.S. approved cancer programs reported that ≈75% of the patients had no demonstrable metastatic tumor at diagnosis of the primary lesion.[1] Hence, of the ≈5,600 newly diagnosed patients with STS per year in the US., there can be expected to be ≈4,200 patients with clinically staged I—IVA disease, nearly all of whom will be sufficiently fit to be candidates for definitive treatment. The value of radiation in the management of these patients is the subject of this chapter.

Radiation Sensitivity of STS Cells In Vitro

The radiation sensitivity of cell lines derived from STS and from squamous cell carcinomas (SCC) of the head and neck region have been assessed in vitro by Wieschelbaum [unpublished data, 1990]. He employed cells in exponential phase, equilibrated with air, single radiation doses, and colony formation as the end point for cell viability. Figure 1 presents the cumulative distribution of the SF2 values for the cells derived from the two types of tumors.[2] The result is an implication that the intrinsic radiation sensitivity of cells of STS is greater than for the cells of squamous cell carcinomas. We do not take these in vitro results as proof that the STS cell in vivo are relatively so sensitive; rather, the data do provide strong support for the idea that radiation can be expected to be approximately equally effective in

---

[1] This survey was limited to patients with sarcoma of soft tissues with these exclusions: age ≤17; anatomic sites-viscera, CNS, nodes; and Kaposi's sarcoma.
[2] SF_2 represents the survival fraction following 2 Gy.

Pinedo, H.M., Verweij, J., and H.D. Suit (eds.): Soft Tissue Sarcomas: New Developments in the Multidisciplinary Approach to Treatment. © *1991 Kluwer Academic Publishers, Boston. ISBN: 0–7923–1139–6. All rights reserved.*

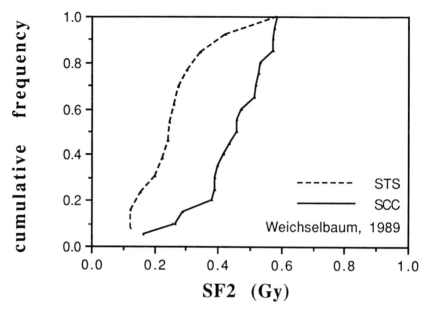

Figure 1. Cumulative distribution of SF2 values for cell lines established from 20 squamous cell carcinomas of the head and neck, and 13 sarcomas of soft tissue (including 1 osteosarcoma). The mean SF2 values are 0.45 ± 0.25 and 0.27 ± 0.35 (± SEM) for the STS and STS, respectively.

the killing of cells of STS as SCC in the patient. There may be micrometabolic environments in vivo that render the STS cells relatively less sensitive than the SCC cells; any such factors would not appear to be of major importance.

Radiation Alone

Radiation is well established as an effective modality in the treatment of patients with STS [2-9]. This is particularly so when radiation is combined with surgery. For those patients who are not operable for medical or technical reasons, radiation has been demonstrated to be a good second line modality. However, successful treatment of these tumors by radiation alone requires that the dose be high (viz., ≥70 Gy) and that the lesion be of modest size. There are numerous accounts of permanent regression of STS following radiation alone [5-9]. The late effects of doses in the range indicated are clinically significant with currently employed techniques; this is especially so for the treatment of large tumors: hence, the desire to employ surgery for the final, or "boost", dose.

Early in the history of radiation therapy, STSs gained a reputation for extraordinary radiation resistance [10]. This was based on several factors:

Table 1. Radiation dose level (TDF) and local control of soft tissue carcinoma when treated by radiation alone.

Dose (TDF)	Tumor size			
	5 cm	5—9 cm	10—14 cm	15 cm
<105	2/2	4/9	2/2	2/3
95—104				0/1
80—94		1/3	0/1	0/3
>80		1/3	0/1	0/1

After Tepper and Suit, 1985 [8].

(1) the sarcomas, with few exceptions, are quite large; (2) treatment was administered by low energy beams with resultant moderate dose levels; (3) tumor regression was slow, especially in comparison with the epithelial tumors of the tonsil, skin, uterine cervix etc.; and (4) long-term control was presumed to be predicted simply by the rate of regression during and/or immediately after the completion of radiation therapy. Thus, the early experiences in radiation therapy for patients with STS were based on large lesions treated to low-modest doses, and the responses judged in terms of the pattern of the prompt regression. Experience with high energy x-ray beams, using high doses, has shown that the observed regressions in the successfully treated lesions are usually quite slow relative to those for the common epithelial tumors. Provided the responses are assessed with respect to long-term freedom from progression, clinical results with modern radiation therapy has shown that these tumors are not characterized by an extraordinary radiation resistance. Our evaluation of current clinical data is that the likelihood of permanent control of tumors of a specified size and treated by a given radiation protocol is approximately the same for epithelial and mesenchymal tumors. Neither epithelial or mesenchymal tumors of, say, ≥65 ml in volume (≥5 cm diameter) are controlled by well-tolerated doses of radiation at a high probability. Local success is highly dependent upon the dose administered and the size of the lesion, as demonstrated by the data given in Table 1. Local failure was the rule in patients receiving less than ≈65 Gy, especially for the larger tumors.

Rationale for Combining Radiation and Surgery

This subject has been considered previously [11,12]. Briefly, the concept is that (1) local excision of STS was replaced by radical wide-field resectional surgery because of the high local failure rate due to the microextension of sarcoma beyond the grossly evident tumor; (2) the consequence was a marked improvement in local control rates, but large volumes of grossly normal tissue were being resected; (3) accordingly, there were major functional and cosmetic deficits; and (4) moderate and readily tolerated radiation

63

doses ($\approx$60 Gy in $\approx$6 weeks) will inactivate the cells constituting the sub-clinical extensions of tumor. Hence, such radiation treatment combined with conservative surgery should achieve a local control result similar to that by radical resection alone, and with greatly improved functional and cosmetic results. The need to resect large volumes of grossly normal tissue in order to secure clear margins would be eliminated. Further, the combined approach would be applicable to a much greater proportion of STS patients; this pertains particularly to patients whose tumors are extracompartmental. Also, some inoperable lesions would become operable. There is a clinically significant advantage of radiation therapy relative to surgery: the treatment volume can be readily designed to encompass major nerves, blood vessels, tendons, etc., which would be encompassed in the surgical specimen only at the price of significant morbidity.

Radiation Therapy Technique

Technical aspects of radiation therapy have been considered in previous papers [13,14]. The basic concepts are (1) to define the target in 3D, using CT, MRI, and other procedures as indicated; (2) to relate the defined target to fiducial markers (bone landmarks or other reasonably fixed structures); (3) in collaboration with clinical physicists, to design a treatment plan that achieves the closest feasible approximation of the treatment volume to the target volume; (4) this plan may use one or more of external photon beams (all of the same energy or of differing energies, with wedge and/or compensator filters), electrons, protons, brachytherapy procedures, and customized and rigid immobilization devices; and (5) to determine the accuracy and precision of the alignment of the target with the beam. As the aim is to distribute the radiation dose in accordance with the likely distribution of tumor clones, there are two and often three treatment volumes, which translates into the "shrinking field" technique. This means that there are several treatment plans. The radiation dose is decided after the total treatment strategy has been decided, viz., timing and scope of surgery, status of normal tissues, if chemotherapy is to be a part of the plan, the treatment volume, and the normal tissues included. For the usual patient condition treated by radiation and surgery, we recommend 50 Gy (2 Gy/fraction) preoperatively, conservative surgery 2.5 weeks later with 16 Gy given intraoperatively by brachytherapy/electron beam or a postoperative boost dose to the tumor bed, as defined by small clips, for a total of 66 Gy. For the patient treated postoperatively, the does is usually 66 Gy, using a shrinking field technique. For patients receiving adriamycin chemotherapy, we reduce the dose per fraction and the total dose by 10%; adriamycin is never given concurrently with radiation. Selection of field dimensions is complex, with major emphasis given to the size and histological grade of the sarcoma. For small and Grade I sarcomas, the margins are usually $\approx$5 cm beyond the limits of the gross lesion. On the other hand, for the large Grade III sarcomas arising in muscle, the margin may be some 15 cm beyond the gross disease. The entity of the muscle is considered to be the target only for rhabdomyosarcoma or where the margins mentioned encompass the entire muscle. These suggested margins are at best guidelines. The definition of the target is a matter of clinical judgment. Except for unusual circumstances, the tumor is not likely to extend into the tendonous origin or insertion. Further, bone, major fascial planes, interosseous membranes, etc. do serve as effective barriers to tumor spread; these structures may be considered as target margins in most situations where imaging studies yield no evidence that they have been transgressed. For postoperative radiation therapy, the surgical bed and all tissues handled surgically are classed as targets.

Local Control of STS Following Modern Treatment Methods

The major treatment approaches to the primary STS employed today are multimodality. These are conservative surgery combined with moderate dose radiation therapy (radiation administered pre- or postoperatively by external beam techniques; intraoperatively by electron beam techniques; intraoperative brachytherapy), and the combined approach of radiation, intra-arterial chemotherapy, and conservative surgery. Less frequently, amputation or radical compartmental resection alone is utilized. The latter has less applicability, as it cannot be applied against tumors that are extra-compartmental, e.g., groin, knee, distal leg, axilla, elbow, distal arm/hand, head/neck, etc. Although high local control rates are obtained by radical surgery in carefully selected patients, there is the inevitable resection of generous amounts of grossly normal tissue in order to obtain truly negative margins. Selected recent 5-year local failure rates by radical surgery alone have been 9% among 103 patients [15] and 14% among 132 patients [16].

Conservative multimodality procedures yield comparable rates, as evident by the data presented in Table 2.

Local success depends heavily upon the size of the tumor for radiation alone, but to a lesser degree for radiation combined with surgery. In our experience, size appears to be a more important parameter for radiation given postoperatively than preoperatively. This is evident from the data presented in Table 3. The local control results were higher in the size groups ≥150 mm for the preoperative than postoperative treatment. This contrasts sharply with the role of sarcoma size on the probability of the development of distant metastasis. In Table 4 are shown the observed frequencies of DM according to tumor size in patients who have local control of their Grade 2 and 3 STS. The DM frequency increased steeply with size, viz., 8% for sarcomas ≤25 mm to 90% for sarcomas >200 mm in diameter. This demonstrates that stratification for size is extremely important in any analysis of disease-free survival.

Table 2. Local failure rate in patients with sarcoma of soft tissue treated by radiation and surgery (± chemotherapy).

Center	No. patients	Local failure (%)	Reference
MGH			
Postop	144	14	Suit, unpublished
Preop	114	9	Suit, unpublished
IGR	89	14	41
RPMI	53	14	42
MDAH			
Postop	253	20.9	43
Preop	110	10	4
NCI	128	10	44
UCSF	29	10	45
U. Florida	19	5	46

Table 3. Five-year actuarial local control results according to size.

| Size (mm) | Postop | | Preop | |
	No. patients	LC (%)	No. patients	LC (%)
≤25	24	88	10	82
26—49	51	91	15	83
50—100	68	84	61	92
101—150	14	92	29	100
151—200	7	54	23	76
>200	3	67	12	100
Total	167	85	150	89

LC = Local control. Suit, unpublished.

Table 4. Five-year actuarial distant metastasis probability in local control patients, as a function of tumor size and grade in MGH series.

| Size (mm) | Grade 1 | | Grade 2 and 3 | |
	No. patients	DM (%)	No. patients	DM (%)
≤25	7	0	24	8
26—50	12	0	47	19
51—100	18	6	98	44
101—150	7	0	35	55
151—200	4	25	19	71
>200	4	0	10	90
Total	52	6	233	41

DM = Distant metastasis. Suit, unpublished.

66

Table 5. Results of treatment of patients with sarcoma of soft tissue by i.a. doxorubicin, radiation, and resection.

Period	Treatment no. patients	Doxorubicin	Radiation	Local failure (%)	Amputation (%)
1972—76	63	−	±	22	33
1974—84	77	+	3.5 Gy × 10	5	4
1981—84	137	+	3.5 Gy × 5	12	5
1984—87	97	+	3.5 Gy × 8	5	2

Eilber et al., 1988 [17].

The combination of radiation, intra-arterial adriamycin, and resection has been found to be an effective approach to these tumors, by Eilber [17]. Their data for four successive time periods are presented in Table 5. The radiation dose was adjusted from 35 to 17.5 to 28 Gy; the latter is currently employed, with an improved balance between tumor control and treatment-related morbidity. The local control results as given are not actuarial, hence, not directly comparable with those for preoperative radiation from the MGH. They do make the point that there are several highly effective strategies for limb salvage therapy.

Local control is important to the long-term survival of the patient. This has most convincingly been demonstrated from studies based on experimental animal tumor systems. For example, investigations on early generation isotransplants of C3H/Sed mouse fibrosarcomas and squamous cell carcinomas [12,18] revealed that local failure was associated with significantly increased rates of distant metastasis (DM). Further, the likelihood of DM was dependent on the size of the recurrent tumor at salvage surgery. An analysis of clinical data of the Institute of Oncology, Warsaw [19], indicated that DM was significantly more likely in patients who failed locally than in local control patients; this result was obtained even though allowance was made for major prognostic variables (e.g., stage of tumor, extent of surgery, etc.). A similar conclusion was reached by Collin et al. [20]. These findings require that efficacy of limb-sparing treatment procedures be continuously monitored in each institution to assure that results are being maintained at the expected level. Further, follow-up examinations need to be at a frequency such that salvage procedures can be implemented for minimal-sized recurrences.

The cosmetic and functional results in patients treated by the various methods cannot be compared on the basis of the available published data. That complications do arise after surgery alone needs to be remembered. This is documented in two recent papers. Complications requiring rehospitalization developed in 10% of the 100 patients subjected to "local excision" at the NCI [21]. At the Memorial Hospital, major complications were scored in 3% of the patients [22]. This was less than the 22% of patients in the surgery-plus-brachytherapy patients. Of the 110 patients treated by preoperative radiation therapy at the M.D. Anderson Hospital, 15 (14%) major complications occurred [4]. Lampert et al. [23] have reviewed the functional status of 40 patients treated at the NCI by surgery and radiation therapy. Virtually all of the severe late changes appeared among patients with sarcomas of the lower extremity (LE). Of 20 patients with LE sarcomas, severe edema, loss of functional capacity, and life style changes developed in 4, 7, and 11, respectively. These results point out that there is a great need to assess the benefit of the extent of the surgery, the radiation field sizes, and the dose levels employed.

The severity of the late tissue changes following the application of radiation and surgery will depend upon these factors: lesion size, lesion site, scope of the surgery (the size of the surgical defect and the extent of the efforts to reduce that defect, viz., vascularized flaps, drainage system, patient immobilization), status of the normal tissues, presence of concomitant systemic diseases (diabetes, hypertension, etc.), radiation dose (total dose, fractionation pattern, field sizes, dose rate), and concomitant chemotherapy (specific drugs, dose, route of administration, normal tissue toxicity of the drugs employed). There is an obvious practical need for prospective evaluations by independent observers of the cosmetic and functional status of patients treated by the several limb-sparing procedures.

Hyperthermia in the Treatment of patients with STS

Hyperthermia is under intensive laboratory and clinical study as an anticancer treatment modality. The rationale for this use of heat is (1) mammalian cells are killed by low levels of heat, viz., ≈40 to 43.5°C is the temperature range often used; (2) the heat/cell survival curve is similar in shape to that for radiation; (3) the age response function for heat inactivation is complimentary to that for radiation, i.e., S phase cells are the most thermally sensitive, whereas S is the most radiation-resistant phase; (4) for a given power input (RF, microwave, ultrasound), tumor tissue often achieves a higher temperature than the surrounding normal tissue because of relatively poor blood flow patterns; (5) some cells of tumor tissue (but not normal tissue) are metabolically deprived and are of increased thermal sensitivity; and (6) heat, at the levels mentioned, sensitizes cells to the killing effects of radiation. Thus, there is a powerful biologic basis for the clinical investigation of hyperthermia alone and in combination with radiation. Unfortunately, the technical means for realizing a known level and an acceptable uniformity of heating in human tissues have been developed for only a few special anatomic situations.

Gillette et al. [24] have studied canines with STS treated by radiation alone (35 to 55 Gy) or combined with hyperthermia (microwave or ultrasound), using 39 to 41.3°C. There was a significantly greater time to regrowth for the combined radiation and 39 to 40°C hyperthermia treatments.

68

Issels et al. [25] have studied 25 human patients with recurrent or progressive STS at various sites treated by regional hyperthermia combined with ifosfamide plus etoposide. Four patients underwent subsequent resection, and no intact cells were found in the specimen; in a fifth patient, there was ≥50% necrosis. Additionally, there were two partial responses, eight no changes, and ten progressions of tumor. These results do constitute evidence for some level of clinical effectiveness. There may well be an important clinical gain for the use of interstitial hyperthermia for those exceptional STSs that are nonresectable, but reasonably accessible for such a technique. At this point our preference is for the use of conservative surgery to remove the grossly evident tumor, where that is feasible.

We posit that conservative surgery is the ultimate "boost", i.e., advantageous over ultra-high dose "boost" photon doses, fast neutrons, hyperthermia, etc. Even so, there are needs for more effective means for the treatment of the nonresectable tumors.

Intraoperative Brachytherapy

There is an expansion of clinical activity in the area of brachytherapy in general. This is also seen in the STS field. Brachytherapy provides the potential of a near optimal dose distribution, as the radiation sources are positioned directly in the tumor; this is aided by the extremely rapid fall-off of dose with distance from the implant. There have been a number of reports of small series of patients treated by this approach [26-31], which provide evidence of the efficacy of this strategy when applied to appropriately selected patients. Brennan et al. [31] have conducted a Phase III trial of surgical resection alone or combined with an ^{192}Ir implant performed intraoperatively. The local failure results were (not actuarial) 4% and 14% for the brachytherapy and the surgery alone groups, respectively. They also pooled the results from their trial patients and patients not in the trial. The results at 30 months were 95% for the brachytherapy group (52 patients) and 83% for the surgery alone group (65 patients). Clearly, this is an effective treatment modality. However, all of the patients were resectable in order to be entered into their study. For the series described earlier for preoperative radiation therapy, some of the patients were nonoperable at the initiation of the radiation, but became operable after the radiation therapy. Thus, the preoperative and the brachytherapy series are not fully comparable in terms of the local extent of disease.

Intraoperative Electron Radiation Therapy

This technique is achieving substantial popularity at this writing because of the ease of augmenting the radiation dose by this seemingly low morbidity procedure. The approach is simple and direct: the radiation sensitive tissues overlying the tumor are packed out of the beam path, and the electron cone positioned onto the exposed tumor or tumor bed. In most institutions, this method is given after the completion of a course of fractionated external beam radiation therapy. The intraoperative dose is usually in the range of 10 to 20 Gy given as a single dose. Willett et al. [32] have employed this strategy in the treatment of 14 patients with primary or recurrent retroperitoneal STSs. In 11 patients for whom the resection of the gross disease was complete and the full dose preoperative and intraoperative radiation was administered, one local failure has been seen to date. Kinsella et al. [33] have compared the morbidity of radical resection of retroperitoneal STS combined with IORT or postoperative radiation therapy. There was an evident reduction in severity of morbidity, but no clear gain in tumor control.

Proton Beam Therapy

Proton beams are of potential value in the radiation therapy of the cancer patient because of the qualitatively different dose distributions achievable with proton beams. This is due to the physical fact that protons are heavy charged particles and as such have a finite range that is dependent upon their energy. Hence, by the utilization of beams with appropriate energy distributions, the treatment volume can be designed to conform more closely to the target volume than is feasible with photons, for certain anatomic sites. This permits a higher radiation dose to the target and accordingly a higher tumor control probability, with a lesser frequency and severity of normal tissue damage. At the Massachusetts General Hospital/Harvard Cyclotron Laboratory, eight patients with STS in the paraspinal tissues treated by conservative excision and postoperative protons had local control with no instance of damage to the cord. Similarly good results have been realized in the treatment of patients with STS overlying the hip, elbow, wrist, and shoulder joints. The gain in these treatments are in the area of reduced morbidity. The total experience is too limited to these special sites to make more general comments.

Fast Neutron Radiation Therapy

Conventional radiation therapy is based on low LET radiations, primarily photons (x-rays and gamma rays) and electrons. These are characterized by LET values of <1 KeV of energy being lost per μm of photon path length, i.e., quite sparsely ionizing. The interest in high LET radiations, such as fast neutrons (FN), lies in the different biological effectiveness, with the potential for a greater differential effect between tumor and normal tissue than obtains for photons (x-rays). The basis for the hopeful expectations are (1) a relatively flat age response function (cell kill is less dependent on the cell position in the cell replication cycle); (2) cell sensitivity is less dependent upon the metabolic status, especially pO2; (3) repair of radiation damage is of smaller magnitude than for low LET radiation. Despite these apparent positive factors, a greater efficacy for fast neutron therapy has been generally accepted only for the locally advanced salivary gland tumors. Laramore et al. [34] reviewed the experience from several centers with FN treatment of STS patients and concluded that there was a greater local control rate of STS by FN than photons. A local control of ≈50% in a series of 50 patients treated by FNs for primary or recurrent STS was reported by Pickering [35]. The local control rate in patients with 5 to 10 cm STSs treated by FNs in the series of Schmitt [36] was 76%. In the Hamburg series, Franke reported that 13 of 17 patients had local control of gross STS treated by FN alone [37]. A definitive assessment of these results is quite difficult, as there are no Phase III trials of FN vs. photons against STS. Nor are there published response data for photons alone and FN alone results, which would permit an assessment of the local control with stratification for tumor size, grade, histological type, and anatomical site. In the photon series reported by Tepper et al. [8], there was a steep dependence of local control probability on sarcoma size and total dose. In addition to the question of local control, there has to be an assessment of the late fibrosis and late tissue atrophy, a known important problem for FN therapy. Hence, at this writing no conclusion as to the relative merits of photon and FN therapy can be drawn.

Negative Pion Therapy

Negative pions are another species of high LET radiations The negative pion is a charged particle (−1); the mass is between that of an electron and a proton; the pion loses energy, as expected for a charged particle, until the energy and velocity is low at near the end of the range, when it interacts with the atomic nucleus of the irradiated material. This interaction causes spallation of the nucleus, with the resultant production of several very high LET particles, e.g., protons, alpha particles, etc. The principal test of negative pions against 27 patients with STS has been at the Paul Scherer Institute (near Zurich), which was reported to have yielded local control in 23 patients; several of those few failures were described as having developed outside of the treatment volume [38]. These various results indicate that a rigorous test of high LET particles vs. photons against sarcomas of the same size and grade is clearly warranted.

Desmoid Tumors

Miralbell et al. [39] reviewed the experience at the MGH with patients who had surgical resection of their primary desmoid tumors, but with positive histological margins, and who were observed only. Among the 21 patients who had grossly complete resection, there have been four regrowths; these four patients have had successful salvage treatment. There were five patients whose surgical resection was not grossly complete; all five regrew. We favor observation only following grossly complete resection of the primary desmoid tumor. Radiation therapy is quite effective in the treatment of the desmoid tumor, viz., a local control rate of ≈80 to 90% following doses of ≈60 Gy in some 6 to 7 weeks [39]. There does not appear to be convincing evidence of greater efficacy for doses greater than the 55 to 60 Gy range. McCullough et al. [40] reported local control for 5 years of two massive desmoids by low doses: 40 Gy to a 20 × 20 cm trapezius lesion and 35 Gy to a 20 cm right upper quadrant tumor. Desmoids are not true sarcomas. They do not metastasize, and the response to various therapeutic regimen is, at present, highly unpredictable. For the patient with an unresectable desmoid (for medical or technical reasons), we favor radiation therapy to a dose of ≈60 Gy. For patients with grossly incomplete resection or recurrent disease, if not resectable with confidence of secure margins, radiation therapy should be considered an an effective option.

References

1. Lawrence W, Jr, Donegan WL, Nachimuth N, et al.: Adult soft tissue sarcomas. A pattern of care survey of the American College of Surgeons. Ann Surg 205:349—359, 1987.
2. Suit HD, Russell WO, Martin RG: Sarcoma of soft tissue: Clinical and histopathologic parameters and response to treatment. Cancer 35:1478—1483, 1975.
3. Suit HD, Mankin HJ, Wood WC, Gebhardt MC, Harmon DC, Rosenberg A, Tepper JE, Rosenthal D: Treatment of the patient with stage M_0 sarcoma of soft tissue. J Clin Oncol 6:854—862, 1988.
4. Barkley HT, Martin RG, Romsdahl MM, Lindberg R, Zagard GK: Treatment of soft tissue sarcomas by preoperative irradiation and conservative surgical resection. Int J Radiat Oncol Biol Phy 14:693—699, 1988.
5. Cade S: Soft tissue tumours: Their natural history and treatment section of surgery. President's Address. Proc R Soc Med 44:19—36, 1951.
6. Windeyer B, Dische S, Mansfield CM: The place of radiotherapy in the management of fibrosarcoma of the soft tissues. Clin Radiol 17:32—40, 1966.
7. McNeer GP et al.: Effectiveness of radiation therapy in management of sarcoma of soft somatic tissues. Cancer 22:391—397, 1968.
8. Tepper JE, Suit HD: Radiation therapy alone for sarcoma of soft tissue. Cancer 56:475—479, 1985.
9. Slater, JD, McNeese MD, Peters LJ: Radiation therapy for unresectable soft tissue sarcomas. Int J Radiat Oncol Biol Phys 12:1729—1734, 1986.
10. Paterson, R: The treatment of malignant disease by radium and x-rays. London: Edward Arnold, 1953.

11. Suit HD, Mankin HJ, Wood WC, Proppe KH: Radiation and surgery in the treatment of primary sarcoma of soft tissue: Pre-operative, intra-operative and post-operative. Franz Buschke Lecture, University of California at San Francisco, March 1982. Cancer 55:2659—2667, 1985.

12. Todoroki T, Suit HD: Therapeutic advantage in pre-operative single dose radiation combined with conservative and radical surgery in different size murine fibrosarcomas. J Surg Oncol 29:207—215, 1985.

13. Suit HD, Rosenberg AE, Harmon DC, Mankin HJ, Wood WC, Rosenthal D: Soft tissue sarcomas. In: Treatment of cancer, 2nd edition. Halnan K, Sikora K (eds). London: Chapman and Hall, pp 657—677, 1990.

14. Suit HD, Mankin HJ, van Groeningen C: Sarcoma of soft tissues. Oxford Textbook of Oncology. Peckham M, Pinedo R, Veronesi U (eds). London: Oxford University Press, in press, 1990.

15. Alvegard TA, Berg NO: Histopathology peer review of high-grade soft tissue sarcoma: The Scandinavian sarcoma group experience. J Clin Oncol 7:1845—1851, 1989.

16. Brennan MF, Hilaris B, Shiu MH, et al.: Local recurrence in adult soft-tissue sarcoma. A randomized trial of brachytherapy. Arch Surg 122:1289—1293, 1987.

17. Eilber FR, Giuliano A, Huth J, Mirra J, Rosen G, Morton D: Neoadjuvant chemotherapy, radiation, and limited surgery for high grade soft tissue sarcoma of the extremity. Recent concepts in sarcoma treatment (Proceedings of the International Symposium on Sarcomas, Tarpon Springs, FL, 1987). Ryan JR, Baker LH (eds). Dordrecht, The Netherlands: Kluwer Academic Publishers, pp 115—122, 1988.

18. Ramsay J, Zietman A, Preffer F, Suit HD: The growth and cell kinetics of a secondary tumor after radiation or surgical treatment of the primary tumor. Int J Radiat Oncol Biol Phys 17:809—813, 1989.

19. Emrich LJ, Ruka W, Driscoll DL, Karakousis CP: The effect of local recurrence on survival time in adult high-grade soft tissue sarcomas. J Clin Epidemiol 42:105—110, 1989.

20. Collin C, Godbold J, Hajdu S, Brennan M: Localized extremity soft tissue sarcoma: An analysis of factors affecting survival. J Clin Oncol 5:601—612, 1987.

21. Skibber JM, Lotz MT, et al.: Limb-sparing surgery for soft tissue sarcomas: Wound related morbidity in patients undergoing wide local excision. Surgery 102:447—452, 1987.

22. Arbeit JM, Hilaris BS, Brennan MF: Wound complications in the multimodality treatment of extremity and superficial truncal sarcomas. J Clin Oncol 5:480—488, 1987.

23. Lampert MH, Gerber LH, Glatstein E, Rosenberg SA, Danoff JV: Soft tissue sarcoma: Functional outcome after wide local excision and radiation therapy. Arch Phys Med Rehabil 65:477—480, 1984.

24. Gillette EL, Gillette SM, Dewhirst MW, Thrall DE, Page RL, Powers BE, Withrow SJ, Rosner G, Wong C, Sim DA: Response of canine soft tissue sarcomas to radiation or radiation plus hyperthermia. Abstracts of Papers for the 38th Annual Meeting of the Radiation Research Society, New Orleans, LA, April 1990, p 50.

25. Issels RD, Prenninger SW, Nagele A, Boehm E, Sauer H, Jauch KW, Denecke H, Berger H, Peter K, Wilmanns W: Ifosfamide plus etoposide combined with regional hyperthermia in patients with locally advanced sarcomas: A phase II study. J Clin Oncol, in press.

26. Collins JE, Paine CH, Ellis F: Treatment of connective tissue sarcomas by local excision followed by radioactive implant. Clin Radiol 27:39—41, 1976.

27. Mills EED, Hering ER: Management of soft tissue tumours by limited surgery combined with tumour bed irradiation using brachytherapy and supplementary teletherapy. Br J Radiol 54:312—317, 1981.

28. Novaes PERS: Interstitial therapy in the management of soft-tissue sarcomas in childhood. Med Pediat Oncol 13:221—224, 1985.

29. Gerbaulet A, Panis X, Flamant F, Chassagne D: Iridium afterloading curietherapy in the treatment of pediatric malignancies. Cancer 56:1274—1279, 1985.

30. Curran WJ, Littman P, Raney RB: Interstitial radiation therapy in the treatment of childhood soft-tissue sarcomas. Int J Radiat Oncol Biol Phys 14:169—174, 1988.

73

31. Brennan MF, Hilaris B, Shiu MH, et al.: Local recurrence in adult soft-tissue sarcoma. A randomized trial of brachytherapy. Arch Surg 122:1289—1293, 1987.
32. Willett CG, Wood WC: unpublished data.
33. Kinsella TJ, Sindelar WF, Lack E, et al.: Preliminary results of a randomized study of adjuvant radiation therapy in resectable adult retroperitoneal soft tissue sarcomas. J Clin Oncol 6:18—25, 1988.
34. Laramore GE, Griffith, JT, Boespflus M, Pelton JG, Griffin T, Griffin BR, Russell KJ, Koh W, Parker RG, Davis LW: Fast neutron radiotherapy for sarcomas of soft tissue, bone, and cartilage. Amer J Clin Oncol 12:320—326, 1989.
35. Pickering DG, Stewart JS, Rampling R, Errington RD, Stamp G, Chia Y: Fast neutron therapy for soft tissue sarcoma. Int J Radiat Oncol Biol Phys 13:1489—1495, 1987.
36. Schmitt G, Furst G, von Essen CF, Scherrer: Neutron and neutron-boost irradiation of soft tissues sarcomas. In: Progress in radio-oncology III. Karcher KH (ed). Proceedings of the Third Meeting on Progress in Radio-Oncology, Vienna, 1986. Published by International Club for Radio-Oncologists, pp 175—183, 1987.
37. Franke HD, Schmidt R: Clinical results after therapy with fast neutrons (DT, 14 McV) since 1976 in Hamburg-Eppendorf. In: Progress in radio-oncology, III. Karcher KH (ed). Proceedings of the Third Meeting on Progress in Radio-Oncology, Vienna, 1986. Published by International Club for Radio-Oncologists, pp 164—174, 1987.
38. Greiner RH, Munkel G, Blattman H, et al.: Conformal radiotherapy for unresectable retroperitoneal soft tissue sarcoma. NCI Workshop, "Potential clinical gains by use of superior radiation dose distributions", April 1989, Int J Radiat Oncol Biol Phys, submitted, 1989.
39. Miralbell R, Suit HD, Mankin HJ, Zuckerberg LR, Stracher MA, Rosenberg AE: Fibromatoses: From postsurgical surveillance to combined surgery and radiation therapy. Int J Radiat Oncol Biol Phys 18:535—540, 1990.
40. McCollough WM, Parsons JT, Million RR, Enneking WF, Springfield DS: Radiation therapy for aggressive fibromatosis: The University of Florida experience, unpublished.
41. Abbatucci JS, Boulier N, deRanieri J, Mandard AM, Tanguy A, Verhnes JC, Lozier JC, Busson A: Local control and survival in soft tissue sarcomas of the limbs, trunk walls and head and neck: A study of 113 cases. Int J Radiat Oncol Biol Phys 12:579—586.
42. Karakousis CP, Emrich LJ, Rao U, Krishnamsetty RM: Feasibility of limb salvage and survival in soft tissue sarcomas. Cancer 56:484—491, 1986.
43. Lindberg RD, Martin RG, Romsdahl MM, Barkley HT: Conservative surgery and postoperative radiotherapy in 300 adults with soft tissue sarcomas. Cancer 47:2391—2397, 1981.
44. Potter DA, Glenn J, Kinsella T, Glatstein E, Lack EE, Restrepo C, White DE, Seipp CA, Wesley R, Rosenberg SA: Patterns of recurrence in patients with high-grade soft tissue sarcomas. J Clin Oncol 3:353—366, 1985.
45. Leibel SA, Tranbaugh RF, Wara WM, Beckstead JH, Bovill EG, Phillips TL: Soft tissue sarcomas of the extremities. Cancer 50:1076—1083, 1982.
46. Enneking WF, McAuliffe JA: Adjunctive preoperative radiation therapy in treatment of soft tissue sarcomas: A preliminary report. Cancer Treat Symp 3:37—42, 1985.

7. Systemic Treatment of Advanced or Metastatic Soft Tissue Sarcomas

Jaap Verweij and Herbert M. Pinedo

Adequate local treatment of soft tissue sarcomas has always been difficult in view of the local recurrence rate of 40 to 80% [1]. Most of these relapses occur within 3 years [2]. The use of sophisticated surgical techniques and the addition of postoperative high-dose radiotherapy have considerably reduced the number of local recurrences in extremity lesions [2-5]. Unfortunately, the inability to apply the required high doses of irradiation precluded a similar decrease in local recurrence in truncal lesions after surgery. Early hematogeneous spreading, most frequently to the lungs, is characteristic for soft tissue sarcomas and apparently can only in part be prevented by optimal local control of the primary tumor. Therefore, distant metastases still occur in a considerable number of patients for whom systemic treatment will be considered. This chapter summarizes the present achievements with systemic treatment of advanced soft tissue sarcomas.

Single-Agent Treatment (Table 1)

Anthracyclines

Doxorubicin (DX) was the first active single agent identified for the treatment of adult soft tissue sarcomas [6]. After the first report, it has been studied in over 1,200 patients [7-9], yielding an overall response rate of 22% in nonpretreated patients and 17% in a small group of pretreated patients [10]. A dose-response relationship has been established for single-agent DX, with doses of 60 mg/m^2 or more producing higher response rates than doses of 50 mg/m^2 or less [11], when the drug is given every 3 to 4 weeks. The intermittent high-dose treatment schedule is generally assumed to be the most effective and is used frequently. However, this schedule introduced the problem of cardiotoxicity and limited the possibilities of combining DX with other myelosuppressive drugs. Therefore, there has been an active search for alternative schedules of DX administration and for less toxic anthracycline analogs. Although previous studies suggested that weekly low-dose DX administration was equally as myelotoxic as one administration of high-dose

Pinedo, H.M., Verweij, J., and H.D. Suit (eds.): Soft Tissue Sarcomas: New Developments in the Multidisciplinary Approach to Treatment. © 1991 Kluwer Academic Publishers, Boston. ISBN: 0–7923–1139–6. All rights reserved.

Table 1. Active single agents.

Drug	Previous chemotherapy	No. of patients	Response rate (8%)		Reference
			Overall	Range	
DX	No	1404	22	15—30	7-9
	Yes	18	17	17	10
IFOS	No	93	24	24—25	34,35
	Yes	211	24	7—65	30-36
DTIC	Yes	95	17	17	28,29

DX every 3 weeks [12,13], a study of the Eastern Cooperative Oncology Group (ECOG) randomizing DX 15 mg/m^2 weekly after an initial loading course, with DX 70 mg/m^2 every 3 weeks and with DX-DTIC (dacarbazine) [8], strongly indicates the opposite. The weekly DX administration resulted in less hematologic toxicity, but induced more stomatitis. Both regimens were equally active (16% and 18% responses, respectively), but this is a disappointing response rate for both.

Another alternative DX administration may be continuous infusion, which is thought to be less cardiotoxic [14]. However, its single-agent activity rate has only been determined in a study using continuous infusion at a rate of 3 mg/m^2/day for 28 to 212 days, and was 17% [15].

One reason that most soft tissue sarcoma patients do not respond to anthracyclines may be an overexpression of P-glycoprotein [16]. P-glycoprotein is a cell-surface glycoprotein involved in the active cellular outward transport of a.o. anthracyclines and is overexpressed in association with the multidrug-resistant (MDR) phenotype. In 6 of 25 patients, this MDR phenotype was found.

The reason for evaluating DX analogs, considered to have a more favorable therapeutic index as compared with the parent drug mainly because of lesser degrees of myelosuppression and cardiac toxicity, is obvious. The results of clinical trials with DX analogs and mitoxantrone are summarized in Table 2. Studies with adequate numbers of patients are as yet limited. The EORTC Soft Tissue and Bone Sarcoma Group evaluated two DX analogs, carminomycin and epirubicin. Both drugs were compared with DX in randomized phase II trials. Importantly, both studies were performed in patients without previous chemotherapy. The response rate (25%) to DX was slightly better than the response rate (18%) to epirubcin, but this difference was statistically not significant [17]. On the other hand, toxicity of epirubicin was significantly less than that of DX, especially with respect to myelosuppression. At higher doses of 100 to 130 mg/m^2, toxicity becomes somewhat marked, but remains acceptable, while the response rate in 32 nonpretreated patients was 19% [18].

The only other study on epirubicin [19] was performed in pretreated

Table 2. Activity of anthracyclines analogs and anthracenediones.

Drug	No. of evaluable patients	No. of responsers			Response rate (%)	Reference
		CR	PR	Total		
Epi-DX	137 (20)	5	17	22	16	17,18
Carminomycin	33 (0)	0	1	1	3	20
Aclarubicin	40 (17)	0	1	1	2	21,22
Esorubicin	20 (1)	0	1	1	5	23
Idarubicin	35 (24)	1	1	2	6	24
Menogaril	21 (21)	0	1	1	5	25
Mitroxantrone	107 (94)	0	1	1	1	26,27

CR = complete remission; PR = partial remission; ( ) = number of patients with prior chemotherapy.

patients. No responses were obtained, which in view of the cross resistance between epirubicin and DX, is not unexpected. The observation that cross resistance between both drugs may occasionally not be complete does not justify the use of epirubicin after resistance to the parent drug. Carminomycin [20] was shown to be inactive, as were Aclarubicin [21,22], Esorubicin [23], Idarubicin [24], and Menogaril [25]. Mitoxantrone, an anthraquinone derivate structurally related to DX, at present has been studied mainly in DX-resistant patients [26,27], with minimal-to-absent antitumor activity, and also did not induce any response in 13 nonpretreated patients [26], making it an uninteresting drug in this tumor type.

DTIC

DTIC is the second drug with single-agent activity. The initial phase II study on this drug resulted in a 17% response rate in 53 patients [28]. Based on this single report, the drug was incorporated into combination chemotherapy. Only recently could the date be confirmed by a phase II study conducted by the EORTC Soft Tissue and Bone Sarcoma Group. Using DTIC at a dose of 1.2 g/m^2 by short-term infusion every 3 weeks, they achieved one complete and six partial remissions in 42 evaluable patients [29], with relatively limited toxicity.

The results obtained by the EORTC for second-line DX and DTIC [10,29], indicate that a truly active drug in soft tissue sarcomas will also be discovered in phase II studies in pretreated patients, although this statement should exclude anthracycline analogs, in view of possible cross resistance.

Ifosfamide

The third active drug in the treatment of soft tissue sarcomas is ifosfamide (IFOS), with activity comparable to that of DX (Table 1) In pretreated patients, the overall response rate was 24% [30-36], while it was the same

Table 3. Activity of other single agents.

Drug	No. of evaluable patients	No. of responsers			Response rate (%)	Reference
		CR	PR	Total		
Trimetrexate	20 (20)	0	3	3	15	37
Cisplatin	62 (36)	1	5	6	10	38,39
Cyclophosphamide	67 (29)	1	4	5	8	35
Methyl-GAG	18 (18)	0	0	0	0	41
Piperazinedione	19 (18)	0	1	1	5	42
Bleomycin	32 (32)	0	0	0	0	43
Chlorozotocin	37 (37)	0	1	1	3	43
MGBG	36 (36)	0	1	1	3	43
Bruceantin	34 (34)	0	0	0	0	43
Diaziquone	31 (31)	0	0	0	0	44
Bisantrene	17 (17)	0	0	0	0	45
Mitomycin	16 (12)	0	1	1	6	46
Homoharringtonine	16 (16)	0	0	0	0	47
TGU	19 (19)	0	0	0	0	48
VP-16	26 (24)	0	1	1	4	49
Fludarabine	40 (40)	0	0	0	0	50,51
MZPES	11 (11)	0	0	0	0	52
MDMS	42 (42)	0	0	0	0	53

CR = complete remission; PR = partial remission; ( ) = number of patients with prior chemotherapy.

in nonpretreated patients [34,35], which is mainly due to the inclusion of the never-confirmed initial data in pretreated patients. Although it has never been tested in a randomized study, the drug given in a daily × 3—5 schedule appears to result in similar response rates to using the 24-hour infusion once every 3 weeks. The optimal total dose of IFOS to be adminis-tered is 5 g/m^2. The results of the two studies in nonpretreated patients are practically identical and offer a firm base for the conclusion that this drug has activity in the treatment of soft tissue sarcomas. Based on all IFOS studies, no single histological subtype has shown a preferential sensitivity for the drug, although it is interesting that four of eight patients with mixed mesodermal sarcomas, included in the EORTC study, responded [36].

Other Cytotoxic Drugs (Table 3)

A variety of established and new antineoplastic agents have been studied. The results of the recently performed phase II studies in advanced soft tissue sarcomas are summarized in Table 3. Of course, almost all of the patients in these trials had been pretreated with standard chemotherapy regimens. With two exceptions, disappointingly low response rates were achieved in all of these studies. As a consequence, these drugs, inactive in pretreated patients, do not warrant testing up front. Without the availability of single-agent data, cyclophosphamide has previously been incorporated into combination chemotherapy regimens. One of the important findings of the EORTC study randomizing IFOS vs. cyclophosphamide was that cyclophosphamide cannot be considered to be a drug with interesting activity [35]. Even using a high dose of 1.5 g/m^2, the EORTC Soft Tissue Bone Sarcoma Group achieved an overall response rate of only 8%.

Trimetrexate at a dose of 6 to 8 mg/m^2/day i.v. days 1 to 5 every 3 weeks was studied by the Canadian Sarcoma group, yielding 3 partial remissions (15%) in 20 evaluable pretreated patients, with moderate toxicity [37].

CDDP (cisplatin) is the only other exception among the drugs listed in Table 3. In a study using CDDP at a dose of 120 mg/m^2 every 3 to 4 weeks [38], no significant antitumor activity was found, with a response rate of only 4% in 26 nonpretreated patients, confirming previous reports. In contrast, a study conducted by the Southwest Oncology Group (SWOG) [39] reported a remarkable response rate of 24% with CDDP at a dose of 40 mg/m^2/day on 5 consecutive days every 4 weeks in pretreated patients. Obviously, while toxicity was substantial, these data have to be confirmed by others before meaningful conclusions can be drawn.

Partly in contrast to the conflicting data in other types of soft tissue sarcoma, mixed mesodermal sarcoma of the uterus appears to be sensitive to CDDP [54,55]. Of note, there were also responders among patients with prior chemotherapy. The relative insensitivity of mixed mesodermal sarcomas of the uterus to DX further distinguishes this disease from other soft tissue sarcomas [56].

Biological Response Modifiers

In the recent literature, only two studies on interferons have been reported. Beta-interferon was evaluated in 20 patients, of whom 15 had received previous chemotherapy. One partial response was observed in a patient with fibrosarcoma [58]. Gamma-interferon was studied in 16 patients with advanced soft tissue sarcomas; 14 patients had received prior chemotherapy. No objective responses were obtained [59]. As for most other tumor types in advanced stages, interferons appear to be of little, if any, benefit to soft tissue sarcoma patients. Incidental observations with interleukin-2 have not shown activity [60].

Combination Chemotherapy

In view of the preliminary efficacy of single-agent DX and DTIC and based upon suggested synergism in preclinical studies, the SWOG initiated a study utilizing DX 60 mg/m^2 on day 1 and DTIC 250 mg/m^2/day on days 1 to 5, repeated every 3 weeks. This regimen is known as ADIC (adriamycin (doxorubicin)-DTIC) [61] and yielded an initial response rate of 42%.

The ECOG has recently performed a randomized trial comparing DX 70 mg/m^2 i.v. bolus on day 1 every 3 weeks; with DX 20 mg/m^2 i.v. bolus on days 1, 2, and 3 and 15 mg/m^2 i.v. bolus on day 8 and weekly thereafter; and with ADIC [8]. This trial thus questioned the influence of the dosing schedule of DX and the value of the addition of DTIC. The resulting activity of the single-agent DX regimens was comparable (18% and 16% responses, respectively), while the addition of DTIC significantly ($p < 0.02$) increased the response rate to 30%, mainly by increasing the number of partial remissions. Unfortunately, the higher response rate of the combination was not reflected in an increased overall survival.

Although gastrointestinal toxicity especially was more evident for the combination than the single-agent DX treatments, this did not result in a lower treatment compliance, indicating that the combination side effects, in general, appear tolerable. The Gynecologic Oncology Group (GOG) performed a quite similar trial in uterine sarcomas [62], comparing DX 60 mg/m^2 on day 1 with the same dose of DX plus DTIC 250 mg/m^2/day on days 1 to 5, treatments given every 3 weeks. The difference in response rate was not significant in this subset of patients, with 13 responses (16%) in 80 DX-treated patients and 16 (24%) in 66 ADIC-treated patients.

The value of adding other drugs to DX was also questioned by several other randomized trials. The ECOG previously studied DX 70 mg/m^2 every 3 weeks, vs. DX 50 mg/m^2 plus cyclophosphamide (CTX, or Cytoxan) 750 mg/m^2 plus vincristine (VCR) 1.4 mg/m^2, all by i.v. bolus on day 1 every 3 weeks, vs. CTX 750 mg/m^2 plus VCR 1.4 mg/m^2 plus actinomycin-D (DACT,or dactinomycin) 0.4 mg/m^2, by i.v. bolus on day 1 every 3 weeks [63]. In a total of 200 patients, response rates were 27%, 19%, and 11%, respectively. The difference between the first and the latter regimen was significant ($p = 0.03$) in terms of response, but not in terms of survival. This study strongly suggests that CTX and VCR do not add activity to DX, while replacing DX with DACT results in significantly decreased activity. Apparently VCR, CTX, and DACT have very limited value in the treatment of soft tissue sarcomas.

The GOG [64] randomized 104 patients with uterine sarcomas, comparing DX 60 mg/m^2 every 3 weeks, with DX 60 mg/m^2 plus CTX 500 mg/m^2 every 3 weeks. Both regimens resulted in a 19% response rate, again indicating that CTX does not add to DX.

The ADIC regimen was tested against the same regimen plus either CTX or DACT in a SWOG study [65]. Patients were randomized to receive DX 60 mg/m^2 on day 1 plus DTIC 250 mg/m^2/day on days 1 to 5 every 3 weeks (the ADIC regimen), or ADIC plus CTX 500 mg/m^2 on day 1 every 3 weeks, or ADIC plus DACT 1.2 mg/m^2 on day 1 every 3 weeks. In 276 evaluable patients, the response rates were not statistically significantly different with 33%, 34%, and 24%, respectively. Also, median durations of response and survival and frequency of toxicities from each of the treatments were equivalent. These data confirm the earlier-mentioned ECOG study indicating the very limited value of CTX and DACT in the treatment of adult soft tissue sarcomas.

By using a different schedule of DTIC administration [66], SWOG tried to lessen toxicity of the ADIC regimen. The regimen consisted a 45-minute infusion of DX 60 mg/m^2 and DTIC 750 mg/m^2 on day 1. Courses were administered at 21-day intervals. With 10 complete and 17 partial remissions in 114 evaluable patients, the overall response rate was 24%. Indeed, this regimen appeared to be very well tolerated, with only moderate myelosuppression and moderate nausea and vomiting.

Preliminary data from a randomized SWOG trial comparing bolus vs. continuous infusion administration of DX and DTIC [67] indicates reduced toxicity with the infusion regimen (104 evaluable patients) as compared with the bolus regimen (112 evaluable patients), while response rates were 22% and 23%, respectively. Since 1972, the SWOG has reported several studies, including the original ADIC regimen. A remarkable observation is the constant decrease in response rate over the years, starting with 42% and presently being 23%. This might be related to the improvement in diagnostic techniques enabling a better evaluation of true responses.

Although the single-agent data generated by the EORTC [35] and the earlier-discussed ECOG, GOG, and SWOG studies on combination chemotherapy regimens [63-65] at the moment do not support the inclusion of CTX in combination chemotherapy regimens, this drug together with VCR was incorporated with ADIC, resulting in the CYVADIC regimen (cyclophosphamide [Cytoxan]-vincristine-Adriamycin [doxorubicin]-DTIC) originally studied in the M.D. Anderson Hospital and afterward adopted by several other groups. The original CYVADIC regimen consisted of CTX 500 mg/m^2 i.v. on day 1, VCR 1.5 mg/m^2 i.v. on days 1 and 5, DX 50 mg/m^2 i.v. on day 1, and DTIC 250 mg/m^2 i.v. on days 1 to 5 [68]. In the initial 125 patients studied, 21 complete remissions (CRs) (17%) and 42 partial remissions (PRs) (34%) were achieved. The median duration was 9.5 months for CR and 7 months for PR. One of the important observations was that the CR rate was much higher in patients <50 years of age than in those >50 [69]. Also, after having treated 331 patients with CYVADIC, the investigators could stress the importance of achieving CR because 21% of those patients have remained disease free for more than 5 years and have been potentially cured by chemotherapy [70]. Finally, patients in PR who could be converted to CR by surgery experienced long-term survival, suggesting cure.

A randomized study of the EORTC [71] compared CYVADIC (CTX 500 mg/m^2 i.v. on day 1, VCR 1.5 mg/m^2 on day 1, and DX 50 mg/m^2/day on days 1 to 5 every 4 weeks), with a schedule alternating VCR/CTX and ADIC in similar doses as used with CYVADIC, at 4-weeks intervals. With CYVADIC, 17% CRs and 21% PRs were achieved in 84 patients, while in the cycling arm a significantly lower response rate of 5% CR and 9% PR was achieved in 78 patients ($p = 0.001$), indicating that DX should be administered every 3 or 4 weeks instead of every 8 weeks. Other studies have confirmed the activity of CYVADIC [72]. The regimen induces nausea

Table 4. Various schedules of DTIC infusion in ADIC and CYVADIC combination chemotherapy.

Regimen	DTIC (days of treatment)	Total DTIC dose (mg/m2)	No. of evaluable patients	Response rate (%)			Reference
				CR	PR	Total	
ADIC	1	750	114	9	15	24	66
	1—5	1250	237	11	24	35	8,61
							62,65
CYVADIC	1	750	135	8	20	28	75
	1—3	1200	60	7	42	49	74
	1—5	1250	314	16	26	42	68-73

and/or vomiting in almost all patients, as well as alopecia. Also, leukocytopenia and thrombocytopenia appear to be substantial, but the regimen nevertheless is considered tolerable. The disadvantage of both the original ADIC and CYVADIC regimens is the necessity of hospitalization. Therefore, shorter schedules have been studied [9,66,74]. The response rates and toxicity of these shortened treatments appear comparable to those of the original regimens (Table 4), but proof from a randomized trial is not available.

After confirmation of the activity of IFOS in soft tissue sarcomas [35], this drug was combined with DX. The Royal Marsden Group treated 50 patients with DX 40 to 60 mg/m^2 i.v. on day 1 plus IFOS 5 to 8 g/m^2 by 24-hour infusion on day 1 with mesna uroprotection [34], with courses repeated every 3 weeks. In 57 evaluable patients, they achieved 6 CRs (11%) and 11 PRs (19%), for an overall response rate of 30%. The optimal doses for the combination appeared to be DX 50 mg/m^2 and IFOS 5 g/m^2. Using that schedule, the EORTC Soft Tissue and Bone Sarcoma Group performed a phase II trial in 178 evaluable patients, achieving 16 CRs (9%) and 47 PRs (26%), for an overall response rate of 35% [75]. Also, other groups [76,77] have used similar regimens achieving similar results (Table 5). A comparable response rate could be achieved by replacing DX with Epirubicin [78].

The major toxicities are leukopenia, nausea, vomiting, and alopecia, all of which are manageable. Recently, the EORTC group completed a randomized trial comparing the DX-IFOS regimen with single-agent DX 75 mg/m^2 i.v. on day 1 every 3 weeks, and with CYVADIC administered 1 day every 3 weeks [9].

At the first analysis, 549 of 716 entered patients were evaluated: 212 in the DX arm, 202 in the DX/IFOS arm, and 135 in the CYVADIC arm. The latter study arm was closed early because of a worse response rate in comparison with the other arms at interim analysis. Curiously, the CYVADIC arm now has the highest response rate, with 28% vs. 27% for DX/IFOS and 24% for DX. However the differences are far from being

Table 5. Combination chemotherapy: Most extensively studied combinations.

Drugs	No. of evaluable patients*	Response rate (%)			Reference
		CR	PR	Total	
DX/DTIC	351	10	21	31	8,61,62,65,66
DX/DTIC/CTX/VCR	509	12	26	38	9,68-74
DX/IFOS	485	7	24	31	9,34,76,77

* Cumulative data.

statistically significant, and the toxicity of the combination chemotherapy exceeded that of single-agent DX.

In general, single-agent treatment with an active drug is as effective as combination chemotherapy, but subset analysis should be awaited as well as long-term follow-up for survival. In view of the fact that CR patients may potentially be cured by chemotherapy [70], it appears important to choose a treatment with the aim at achieving CR.

Than still combination chemotherapy appears superior. With the conclusion that DX, IFOS, and DTIC are the only active single agents in the treatment of soft tissue sarcomas, it seems logical to combine these three drugs. At the Dana Farber Cancer Institute, a study with DX 60 mg/m^2, DTIC 900 mg/m^2, and IFOS 7500 mg/m^2, all given together as a 72-hour continuous infusion every 3 weeks, was performed in 62 evaluable patients [79], yielding 6 CRs (10%) and 26 PRs (42%) and acceptable toxicity. However, a Canadian study using slightly lower doses yielded a response rate of only 25% [80].

Prognostic Factors

With several study reports available that deal with the three major combination chemotherapy regimens that appear to be comparable as far as response rates are concerned, it becomes possible to obtain further insight into factors predicting the outcome of chemotherapy. Regarding several factors with a possible influence on the achievement of response, there is certainly no consensus on age, sex, and bone marrow reserve. The most important prognostic factor for response appears to be the performance score [8,69,71,72], which may be partly related to a favorable influence of a <5% weight loss [8]. Although several authors indicate that some tumor types may be more responsive than others (Table 6), combining all data of studies with ADIC-based regimens indicates the opposite. There is no evidence of one histological subtype with a better prognosis.

Another important observation concerns the time required to achieve response. The median time varies from 7 to 10 weeks [8,62,68,72,72], but it

83

Table 6. Response rates in histological subtypes of soft tissue sarcomas.

	Regimen																
	ADIC						CYVADIC									Total	
	[8][a]		[65]		[66]		[68]		[71]		[72]		[74]				
Histology	n[b]	(%)[c]	n	(%)	n	(%)	n	(%)	n	(%)	n	(%)	n	(%)		n	(%)
Leiomyosarcoma	27	(44)	73	(33)	27	(19)	31	(58)	35	(20)	18	(22)	6	(17)		217	(33)
MFH	24	(25)	43	(21)	13	(54)	—		29	(34)	5	(40)	6	(67)		120	(32)
Schwannoma	9	(22)	—		—		—		—		—		2	(50)		11	(27)
Liposarcoma	7	(14)	16	(19)	—		12	(41)	15	(33)	5	(40)	4	(25)		59	(29)
Fibrosarcoma	4	(0)	—		6	(50)	21	(48)	19	(37)	2	(50)	9	(56)		61	(43)
Synoviasarcoma	3	(0)	10	(33)	2	(0)	2	(50)	7	(28)	—		9	(67)		30	(33)
Angiosarcoma	—		12	(25)	—		5	(60)	7	(14)	—		—			26	(26)
Neurosarcoma	—		12	(33)	10	(20)	13	(69)	6	(17)	—		—			41	(39)
Rhabdomyosarcoma	—		14	(29)	8	(25)	13	(54)	4	(25)	5	(40)	9	(44)		53	(38)

[a] [ ] = reference.
[b] n = number of evaluable patients.
[c] (%) = response rate.

is even more important to realize that treatment periods as long as 32 [68], 56 [8], or 101 [71] weeks may be required to achieve response, indicating that soft tissue sarcomas respond rather slowly to chemotherapy.

Mixed Mesodermal Sarcomas

As has been indicated, cisplatin (CDDP, or cisdiamminedichloroplatin) can be considered a modestly active single agent for the treatment of soft tissue sarcomas, which has been confirmed by the absence of an additive effect of CDDP when combined with active drugs [73,81-84]. In contrast to these general data, mixed mesodermal sarcomas (MMS) appear to respond to some extent to CDDP. In a phase II trial with single-agent CDDP at a dose of 50 mg/m^2 every 3 weeks as second-line chemotherapy, five of 28 (18%) patients achieved a response [54], and at a higher dose, Gershenson et al. even achieved a 28% response rate [55]. These data in MMS appear to be confirmed by limited data on combination chemotherapy including CDDP, achieving 3 responses (27%) in 11 patients. Although DX appears to be less active in MMS than in other histological subtypes [56,57], others have combined DX and CDDP. Seltzer et al. [85] applied 50 mg/m^2 DX plus 50 mg/m^2 CDDP both i.v. on day 1 every 3 weeks, achieving 3 CRs and 2 PRs in 6 patients. The Toronto group [86] treated 15 patients with MMS of the ovary with either CAP [CTX, Adriamycin (DX), and Platinol (CDDP)] or CYVADIC, achieving a 60% response rate. Jansen et al. [87] achieved five remissions in six patients, with a combination of cyclophosphamide, hexamethylmelamine, doxorubicin, and cisplatin (CHAP-5). Of course, for the latter two studies, we should also consider the possible role of CTX because this drug may also be active in MMS [35]. In the near future, the role of CDDP as well as CTX in this rare, but less-DX responsive, sarcoma subtype should be explored.

Induction Chemotherapy

The value of preoperative chemotherapy in the treatment of locally far-advanced soft tissue sarcomas is one of the important issues of investigation in the present decade.

Intra-arterial chemotherapy is discussed elsewhere in this book. However, Rouesse et al. [88] recently reported a series of 34 patients with locally far-advanced, but nonmetastatic, sarcomas treated with either DX-CTX-CDDP-DTIC-vindesine (DCPAV), CYVADIC, or DX-IFOS, achieving 38% remissions; 24 patients underwent surgery after 2 to 7 cycles of chemotherapy, which in 12 proved to be radical. Patients who did not undergo radical operation were irradiated postoperatively. While 2-year survival was only 18% in those patients who never achieved CR, it was 80%

in patients who achieved CR after chemotherapy plus surgery plus radiotherapy, a figure at least suggesting a benefit of preoperative systemic chemotherapy. Also, from other groups using doxorubicin-based chemotherapy, high response rates and even higher resectability rates were reported [79,89]. Clearly this type of treatment should be further explored in randomized trials.

Conclusion

The last few years have shown a trend toward consensus in the chemotherapeutic approach to soft tissue sarcomas. Three active single agents (DX, IFOS, and DTIC) are available. CTX and CDDP may also be considered active in the treatment of mixcd mesodermal sarcomas. At this moment, there is no proof that combination chemotherapy yields higher response rates or improved survival when compared with single-agent treatment, although this general statement may not apply for all subsets, and combination chemotherapy on the contrary does yield higher complete remission rates, which may be important because of indications that these patients may potentially be cured. Although it is not clear which combination chemotherapy is the best, three regimens emerge as most interesting: ADIC, CYVADIC, and DX-IFOS. The future years will highlight investigations on the combination DX-IFOS-DTIC as well as other high-dose chemotherapy regimens supported by growth factors. The role of systemic preoperative chemotherapy will also have to be further outlined because preliminary data indicate high response rates. However, regarding this topic, survival will be more important than response. Clearly there is still a need for new active drugs, and therefore, the continuous search through phase II trials should be encouraged.

References

1. Enneking WF, Spanier SS, Malawer MM: The effect of the anatomic setting on the results of surgical procedures for soft-part sarcomas of the thigh. Cancer 47:1005—1022, 1981.
2. Lindberg RD, Martin RG, Ramsdahl MM: Surgery and postoperative radiotherapy in the treatment of soft tissue sarcomas in adults. AJR Ther Nucl Med 123:123—129, 1975.
3. Gerson R, Shiu MH, Hajdu SI: Sarcoma of the buttock: A trend toward limb-salvage resection. J Surg Oncol 19:238—242, 1982.
4. Leibel SA, Tranbaugh RF, Wara WM, et al.: Soft tissue sarcomas of the extremities: Survival and patterns of failure with conservative surgery and postoperative irradiation compared to surgery alone. Cancer 50:1076—1083, 1982.
5. Suit HD, Mankin HJ, Wood WC, Proppe KH: Preoperative, intraoperative, and postoperative radiation in the treatment of primary soft tissue sarcoma. Cancer 55:2659—2667, 1985.
6. Bonadonna G, Beretta G, Tanchini G, et al.: Adriamycin (NSC-123127) studies at the Instituto Nazionale Tumori, Milan. Cancer Chemother Rep 6:231—245, 1975.

7. Verweij J, van Oosterom AT, Pinedo HM: Melanomas, soft tissue and bone sarcomas. Eur J Cancer Clin Oncol 4 (Suppl):75—85, 1985.
8. Borden EC, Amato DA, Rosenbaum Ch, et al.: Randomized comparison of three adriamycin regiments for metastatic soft tissue sarcomas. J Clin Oncol 5:840—850, 1987.
9. Santoro A, Rouëssé J, Steward W, Mouridsen H, Verweij J, Somers R, Blackledge G, Buesa J, Sayer J, Casali P, Thomas D, Sylvester R: A randomized EORTC phase III study comparing adriamycin vs A plus ifosfamide vs CYVADIC in advanced soft tissue sarcoma. Proc ECCO 5:438, 1989.
10. Blackledge G, van Oosterom A, Mouridsen H, Steward WP, Buesa J, Thomas D, Sylvester R, Rouëssé J: Doxorubicin in relapsed soft tissue sarcoma: Justification of phase II evaluation of new drugs in this disease. An EORTC Soft Tissue and Bone Sarcoma Group study. Eur J Cancer Clin Oncol, in press.
11. O'Bryan RM, Luce JK, Talley RW: Phase II evaluation of adriamycin in human neoplasma. Cancer 32:1—8, 1973.
12. Mitts DL, Gerhardt H, Armstrong D, et al.: Chemotherapy for advanced soft tissue sarcomas: Results of phase I and II cooperative studies. Tex Med 75:43—47, 1979.
13. Chlebowski RT, Paroly WS, Pugh RP: Adriamycin given as a weekly schedule without a loading course: Clinically effective with reduced incidence of cardiotoxicity. Cancer Treat Rep 64:49—51, 1980.
14. Benjamin RS, Yap BS: Infusion chemotherapy for soft tissue sarcomas. In: Soft tissue sarcomas. Baker LH (ed). Boston: Martinus Nijhoff, pp 109—116, 1983.
15. Samuels BL, Vogelzang NJ, Ruane M, Simon MA: Continuous venous infusion of doxorubicin in advanced sarcomas. Cancer Treat Rep 71:971—972, 1987.
16. Gerlach JH, Bell DR, Karakousis C, et al.: P-glycoprotein in human sarcoma: Evidence for multidrug resistance. J Clin Oncol 5:1452—1460, 1987.
17. Mouridsen HT, Bastholt L, Somers R, Santoro A, Bramwell V, Mulder JH, van Oosterom AT, Buesa J, Pinedo HM, Thomas D, Sylvester R: Adriamycin versus epirubicin in advanced soft tissue sarcomas: A randomized phase II/phase III study of the EORTC Soft Tissue and Bone Sarcoma Group. Eur J Cancer Clin Oncol 23:1477—1483, 1987.
18. Chevallier B, Monteuquet PH, Fachini T, Bui B, Tanguy A, Kerbrat P, Bastit PH, Hurteloup P: Phase II study of epirubicin in advanced soft tissue sarcoma. Proc Am Soc Clin Oncol 8:323, 1988.
19. Bodey GP, Yap BS, Ajani J: Clinical trials of 4'epidoxorubicin. Proc 13th Int Congr Chemother 215:23—26, 1983.
20. Bramwell VHC, Mouridsen HT, Mulder JH, Somers R, van Oosterom AT, Santoro A, Thomas D, Sylvester R, Markham D: Carminomycin vs adriamycin in advanced soft tissue sarcomas: An EORTC randomized phase II study. Eur J Cancer Clin Oncol 19:1097—1104, 1983.
21. Bertrand M, Multhauf P, Bartolucci A, Ellison D, Gockerman J: Phase II study of aclarubicin in previously untreated patients with advanced soft tissue sarcoma: A South-Eastern Cancer Study Group trial. Cancer Treat Rep 69:725—726, 1985.
22. Pazdur R, Samson MK, Baker LH: Aclacinomycin: Phase II evaluation in advanced soft tissue sarcoma. Am J Clin Oncol 10:237—239, 1987.
23. Raymond V, Magill GB, Wissel PS, Cheng WE, Ochoa M, Young CW: Phase II trial of deoxydoxorubicin in patients with soft tissue sarcoma. Proc Am Soc Clin Oncol 5:146, 1986.
24. Wissel PS, Magill GB, Raymond V, Well S, Sordillo P, Cheng E: 4'Demethoxydaunorubicin in advanced soft tissue sarcomas: An update with emphasis on patients without prior doxorubicin. Proc Am Soc Clin Oncol 3:259, 1984.
25. Buckner JC, Edmonson JH, Ingle JN, Schaid DJ: Evaluation of menogaril in patients with metastatic sarcomas and no prior chemotherapy exposure. Am J Clin Oncol 12:384—386, 1989.
26. Presant CA, Gans R, Bartolucci AA: Treatment of metastatic sarcomas with mitoxantrone. Cancer Treat Rep 68:813—814, 1984.

27. Bull FE, von Hoff DD, Balcerzak SP, Stephens RL, Panetierre FJ: Phase II trial of mitoxantrone in advanced sarcomas: a South-West Oncology Group study. Cancer Treat Rep 69:231—233, 1985.
28. Gottlieb JA, Benjamin RS, Baker LH, et al.: Role of DTIC (NSC-45338) in the chemotherapy of sarcomas. Cancer Treat Rep 60:199—203, 1976.
29. Buesa J, Mouridsen H, van Oosterom AT, Steward WT, Verweij J, Thomas D: High-dose DTIC in advanced soft tissue sarcoma of the adult: A phase II study of the EORTC Soft Tissue and Bone Sarcoma Group. Proc ECCO 4:235, 1987.
30. Hoefer–Janker H, Scheef W, Gunther U, et al.: Erfahrungen mit der fraktionierten Ifosfamid-Stoss Therapie bei generalisierten malignen Tumoren. Med Welt 26:972—979, 1977.
31. Klein HO, Wickramanayake PD, Coerper CL, et al.: High-dose ifosfamide and mesna as continuous infusion over five days: A phase I/II trial. Cancer Treat Rev 10:167—173, 1983.
32. Czownicki A, Utracka–Hutka B: Contribution to the treatment of malignant tumours with ifosfamide. In: Proceedings of the international Holoxan symposium. Burkert H, Voight HC (eds). Dusseldorf: ASTA-Werke, pp 109—111, 1977.
33. Antman KM, Montella D, Rosenbaum CH, Schwen M: Phase II trial of ifosfamide with mesna in previously treated metastatic sarcoma. Cancer Treat Rep 68:499—504, 1985.
34. Wiltshaw E, Westburg G, Harmer C, McKinna A, Fisher C: Ifosfamide plus mesna with and without adriamycin in soft tissue sarcoma. Cancer Chemother Pharmacol 18 (Suppl 2):S10—12, 1986.
35. Bramwell VHC, Mouridsen H, Santoro A, Blackledge G, Somers R, Verweij J, Dombernowsky P, Onsrud M, Thomas D, Sylvester R, van Oosterom AT: Cyclophosphamide versus ifosfamide: Final report of a randomized phase II trial in adult soft tissue sarcomas. Eur J Cancer Clin Oncol 23:311—321, 1987.
36. Legha S, Papadopoulos N, Usakewicz J, Fenoglio C, Nicaise C, Benjamin R: Role of ifosfamide in the treatment of refractory sarcomas and an evaluation of N-acetylcysteine as a uroprotector. Proc Am Soc Clin Oncol 9:322, 1989.
37. Quirt I, Eisenhauer E, Knowling M, Warr D, Bramwell V, Rusthoven J, Wierzbicki R, Verna S: A phase II study of Trimetrexate in metastatic soft tissue sarcoma. Proc Am Soc Clin Oncol 7:275, 1988.
38. Sordillo PP, Magill GB, Brenner J, Cheng EW, Dosik M, Yagoda A: A phase II evaluation of cisplatin in previously untreated patients with soft tissue sarcomas. Cancer 59:884—886, 1987.
39. Budd GT, Balcerzak S, Mortimer J, Fletcher W: SWOG 8465: High-dose cisplatin for advanced sarcomas. Proc Am Soc Clin Oncol 6:137, 1987.
40. Thigpen JT, Blessing JA, Wilbanks GD: Cisplatin as second-line chemotherapy in the treatment of advanced or recurrent leiomyosarcoma of the uterus: A phase II trial of the Gynecologic Oncology Group. Am J Clin Oncol (CCT) 9:18—20, 1986.
41. Sordillo PP, Magill GB, Welt S: Phase II trial of methylglyoxal-bis guanylhydrazone (methyl-GAG) in patients with soft-tissue sarcomas. Am J Clin Oncol (CCT) 8:316—318, 1985.
42. Thigpen JT, Blessing JA, Homesley HD, Hacker N, Curry SL: Phase II trial of piperazinedione in patients with advanced or recurrent uterine sarcoma: A Gynecologic Oncology Group study. Am J Clin Oncol (CCT) 8:350—352, 1985.
43. Amato Da, Borden EC, Shiraki M, Enterline HT, Rosenbaum C, Davis HL, Paul AR, Stevens CM, Lerner HJ: Evaluation of bleomycin, chlorozotocin, MGBG, and bruceantin in patients with advanced soft tissue sarcoma, bone sarcoma, and mesothelioma. Invest New Drugs 3:397—401, 1985.
44. Chan C, Bartolucci A, Brenner D, Presant C, Davila E, Carpenter J, Greco A, Clamon G, Moore J: Phase II trial of diaziquone in anthracycline-resistant adult soft tissue and bone sarcoma patients: A South-Eastern Cancer Study Group trial. Cancer Treat Rep 70:427—428, 1986.

45. Cowan JD, Gehan E, Rivkin SE, Jones SE: Phase II trial of bisantrene in patients with advanced sarcoma: A South-West Oncology Group study. Cancer Treat Rep 70:685—686, 1986.
46. Wissel P, Magill G, Sordillo P, Cheng E, Hakes T, Applewhite A: A phase II trial of mitomycin C in advanced soft tissue sarcomas. Proc Am Soc Clin Oncol 5:146, 1986.
47. Ajani JA, Dimery I, Chawla SP, Pinnamaneni K, Benjamin RS, Legha S, Krakoff IH: Phase II studies of homoharringtonine in patients with advanced malignant melanomas, sarcoma, and head and neck, breast and colorectal carcinomas. Cancer Treat Rep 70:375—379, 1986.
48. Rouëssé JG, van Oosterom AT, Capellaere P, Kerbrat P, van Groeningen CJ, Thomas D, Benshahar D: Phase II study of 1,2,4-triglycidyl urasol (TGU) in advanced soft tissue sarcoma: A trial of the EORTC Soft Tissue and Bone Sarcoma Cooperative Group. Eur J Cancer Clin Oncol 23:1413—1414, 1987.
49. Dombernowsky P, Buesa J, Pinedo HM, Santoro A, Mouridsen HT, Somers R, Bramwell V, Onsrud M, Rouëssé J, Thomas D, Sylvester R: VP-16 in advanced soft tissue sarcoma: A phase II study of the EORTC Soft Tissue and Bone Sarcoma Group. Eur J Cancer Clin Oncol 23:579—580, 1987.
50. Zalupski M, Pazdur R, Samson M, Baker L: Phase II clinical evaluation of fludarabine in soft tissue and osteosarcomas. Proc Am Soc Clin Oncol 6:135, 1987.
51. Pazdur R, Samson MK, Baker L: Fludarabine phosphate; Phase II evaluation in advanced soft tissue sarcomas. Am J Clin Oncol 10:341—343, 1987.
52. Blackledge G, Verweij J, Füchs R, Keizer J, Rodenhuis C, Rankin E, Kerbrat P, van Oosterom A, Sylvester R, Thomas D and Rouëssé J: A phase II study of M-azido-pyrimethamine ethane sulphonate (MZPES) in advanced recurrent soft tissue sarcoma: An EORTC Soft Tissue and Bone Sarcoma Group study. Eur J Cancer Clin Oncol, in press.
53. Steward WP, Mouridsen HT, Kerbrat P, Somers R, Verweij J, van Oosterom AT, Blackledge G, Thomas D, Sylvester R: Phase II trial of methylene-dimethane sulphonate (MDMS) in advanced soft tissue sarcomas of the adult. Eur J Cancer Clin Oncol 25:1251—1253, 1989.
54. Thigpen JT, Blessing JA, Orr JW, DiSaia J: Phase II trial of cisplatin in the treatment of patients with advanced or recurrent mixed mesodermal sarcomas of the uterus: A gynecologic Oncology Group study. Cancer Treat Rep 70:271—271, 1986.
55. Gershenson DM, Kavanagh JJ, Copeland LJ, Edwardo CL, Stringer CA, Wharton JT: Cisplatin therapy for disseminated mixed mesodermal sarcoma of the uterus. J Clin Oncol 5:618—621, 1987.
56. Morrow CP, Bundy BN, Hoffman J, Sutton G, Homesley H: Adriamycin chemotherapy for malignant mixed mesodermal tumor of the uterus. Am J Clin Oncol (CCT) 9:24—26, 1986.
57. Gershenson DM, Kavanagh JJ, Copeland LJ, Edwards CL, Freedman RS, Wharton JT: High-dose doxorubicin infusion therapy for disseminated mixed mesodermal sarcoma of the uterus. Cancer 59:1264—1267, 1987.
58. Harris J, Das Gupta T, Vogelzang N, Badrinath K, Bonomi P, Desser R, Locker G, Blough R, Johnson C: Treatment of soft tissue sarcoma with fibroblast interferon (beta-interferon): An American Cancer Society/Illinois Cancer Council study. Cancer Treat Rep 70:293—294, 1986.
59. Edmonson JH, Long HJ, Creagan ET, Frytak S, Sherwin SA, Chang MN: Phase II study of recombinant gamma-interferon in patients with advanced non-osseous sarcomas. Cancer Treat Rep 71:211—213, 1987.
60. Salem P, Zikiwski A, Benjamin RS, Wallace S, Levitt D, Mavligit G: Arterial infusion of interleukin-2 for treatment of hepatic metastases from GI leiomyosarcoma: Predisposition to hypersensitivity to iodine-containing media. Proc Am Soc Clin Oncol 8:322, 1989.
61. Gottlieb JA, Baker LH, Quagliana JM, Luce JK, Whitecar JP, Sinkovics JG, Rivkin SE, Brownlee R, Frei E: Chemotherapy of sarcomas with a combination of adriamycin and dimethyl triazeno imidazole carboxamide. Cancer 30:1632—1638, 1972.

89

62. Omura GA, Major FJ, Blessing JA, Sedlacek TV, Thigpen JT, Creasman WT, Zaino RJ: A randomized study of adriamycin with and without dimethyl triazenoimidazole carboxamide in advanced uterine sarcomas. Cancer 52:626—632, 1983.
63. Schoenfeld DA, Rosenbaum CH, Horton J, Wolter JM, Falkson G, De Conti RC: A comparison of adriamycin versus vincristine and adriamycin and cyclophosphamide versus vincristine, actinomycin-D and cyclosphosphamide for advanced sarcoma. Cancer 50: 2757—2762, 1982.
64. Muss HB, Bundy B, DiSaia PJ, Homesley HD, Fowler WC, Creasman W, Yordan E: Treatment of recurrent or advanced uterine sarcoma: A randomized trial of doxorubicin versus doxorubicin and cyclophosphamide (a phase III trial of the Gynecologic Oncology Group). Cancer 55:1648—1653, 1985.
65. Baker LH, Frank J, Fine G, Balcerak SP, Stephens RL, Stuckey WJ, Rivkin S, Saiki J, Ward JH: Combination chemotherapy using adriamycin, DTIC, cyclophosphamide and actinomycin-D for advanced soft tissue sarcomas: A randomized comparative trial — a phase III Southwest Oncology Group study (7613). J Clin Oncol 5:851—861, 1987.
66. Saiki JH, Baker LH, Rivkin SE, Shahbender S, Fletcher WS, Athens JW, Balcerak SP, Bonnet JD: A useful high-dose intermittent schedule of adriamycin and DTIC in the treatment of advanced sarcomas. Cancer 58:2196—2197, 1986.
67. Baker LH, Green S, Ryan J, Rosenberg B, Balcerak S: SWOG 8024: Combined modality therapy for disseminated soft tissue sarcoma, phase III. Proc Am Soc Clin Oncol 6:138, 1987.
68. Yap BS, Baker LH, Sinkovics JG, Rivkin SE, Bottomley R, Thigpen T, Burgess MA, Benjamin RS, Bodey GP: Cyclophosphamide, vincristine, adriamycin and DTIC (CYVADIC) combination chemotherapy for the treatment of advanced sarcomas. Cancer Treat Rep 64:93—98, 1980.
69. Yap BS, Burgess MA, Sinkovics JG, Benjamin RS, Bodey GP: A 5-year experience with cyclophosphamide, vincristine, adriamycin and DTIC (CYVADIC) chemotherapy in 169 adults with advanced soft tissue sarcoma. Proc Am Soc Clin Oncol 22:534, 1981.
70. Yap BS, Sinkovics JG, Burgess MA, Benjamin RS, Bodey GP: The curability of advanced soft tissue sarcomas in adults with chemotherapy. Proc Am Soc Clin Oncol 2:239, 1983.
71. Pinedo HM, Bramwell VHC, Mouridsen H, Somers R, Vendrik CPJ, Santoro A, Buesa J, Wagener TH, van Oosterom AT, van Unnik JAM, Sylvester R, de Pauw M, Thomas D, Bonadonna G: CYVADIC in advanced soft tissue sarcoma: A randomized study comparing two schedules. Cancer 53:1825—1832, 1984.
72. Karakousis CP, Rao U, Park HG: Combination chemotherapy (CYVADIC) in metastatic soft tissue sarcomas. Eur J Cancer Clin Oncol 18:33—36, 1982.
73. Kerzel W, Köning HJ, Walter M, Arnold I: Zytostatische Kombinationsbehandlung fortgeschrittener Sarkome: Ergebnisse einer prospektiv angelegten Studie. Tumor Diagn Ther 6:180—184, 1985.
74. Bui NB, Chauvergne J, Hocke C, Durand M, Brunet R, Coindre JM: Analysis of a series of sixty soft tissue sarcomas in adults treated with a cyclophosphamide-vincristine-adriamycin-dacarbazine (CYVADIC) combination. Cancer Chemother Pharmacol 15:82—85, 1985.
75. Schuette J, Mouridsen H, Santoro A, Steward W, van Oosterom AT, Somers R, Blackledge G, Verweij J, Rouëssé J, Green JA, Pinedo HM, Kaye SB, Kerbrat H, Wagener T, Thomas D, Sylvester R: Adriamycin and ifosfamide, a new effective combination in advanced soft tissue sarcoma. Proc ECCO 4:232, 1987.
76. Cantwell BMJ, Carmichael J, Ghani S, Harris AL: A phase II study of ifosfamide/mesna with doxorubicin for adult soft tissue sarcoma. Cancer Chemother Pharmacol 21:49—52, 1988.
77. Loehrer PJ, Sledge GW, Nicaise C, Usakewicz J, Hainsworth JD, Martelo OJ, Omura G, Braun TJ: Ifosfamide plus doxuribicin in metastatic adult sarcomas: A multi-institutional phase II trial. J Clin Oncol 7:1655—1659, 1989.

90

78. Frustaci S, Foladore S, Lo Re G, Fosser V, Nascimben O, Tuveri G, Magri MD, Monfardini S: Full doses of ifosfamide and epirubicin in advanced soft tissue sarcomas. Proc Am Soc Clin Oncol 8:319, 1989.
79. Elias AD, Ryan L, Aisner J, Antman KH: Doxorubicin, ifosfamide and DTIC (AID) for advanced untreated sarcomas. Proc Am Soc Clin Oncol 6:134, 1987.
80. Bramwell V, Quirt I, Warr D, Verma S, Young V, Knowling M, Eisenhauer E: Combination chemotherapy with doxorubicin, dacarbazine and ifosfamide in advanced adult soft tissue sarcoma. J Natl Cancer Inst 81:1496—1499, 1989.
81. Klippstein TH, Mitrou PS, Kochendörfer KJ, Bergmann L: High dose adriamycin and cisplatinum in advanced soft tissue sarcomas and invasive thymomas: A pilot study. Cancer Chemother Pharmacol 13:78—81, 1984.
82. Hartlapp JH, Munch HJ, Illinger HJ, Wolter H, Jensen JC: Alternatives to CYVADIC combination therapy of soft tissue sarcomas. Cancer Chemother Pharmacol 18 (Suppl 2): S20—S23, 1986.
83. Edmonson JH, Hahn RG, Schutt AJ, Bisel HF, Ingle JN: Cyclophosphamide, doxorubicin and cisplatin combined in the treatment of advanced sarcomas. Med Pediatr Oncol 11: 319—321, 1983.
84. Piver MS, Lele SB, Patsner B: Cisdiamminedichloro-platinum plus dimethyl-triazenoimidazole carboxamide as second- and third-line chemotherapy for sarcomas of the female pelvis. Gynecol Oncol 23:371—375, 1983.
85. Seltzer V, Kaplan B, Vogl S, Spitzer M: Doxorubicin and cisplatin in the treatment of advanced mixed mesodermal uterine sarcoma. Cancer Treat Rep 68:1389—1390, 1984.
86. Moore N, Fine S, Sturgeon J: Malignant mixed mesodermal tumors of the ovary: The Princess Margaret Hospital experience. Proc Am Soc Clin Oncol 5:114, 1986.
87. Jansen RLH, van der Burg MEL, Verweij J, Stoter G: Cyclophosphamide, hexamethylmelamine, adriamycin and cisplatin combination chemotherapy in mixed mesodermal sarcoma of the female genital tract. Eur J Cancer Clin Oncol 23:1131—1133, 1987.
88. Rouëssé JG, Friedman S, Sevin DM, Le Chevalier TH, Spielmann ML, Contesso G, Sarrazin DM, Genin JR: Preoperative induction chemotherapy in the treatment of locally advanced soft tissue sarcomas. Cancer 60:296—300, 1987.
89. Lagarde C, Bui NB, Marée D, Coindre JP, Kantor G, Bussières E: Locally advanced soft tissue sarcomas. Preliminary results of a multi-disciplinary approach with initial (neo-adjuvant) chemotherapy in a series of 46 patients. Proc Am Soc Clin Oncol 7:274, 1988.

8. Adjuvant Chemotherapy for Soft Tissue Sarcomas

Wilson C. Mertens and Vivien H.C. Bramwell

Introduction

Many patients presenting with soft tissue sarcoma have a poor prognosis as a consequence of the tendency of these tumours to invade extensively, recur locally, and metastasize hematogenously early in the course of the disease. Nevertheless most patients present without clinically evident metastases, and gains in survival will derive from improved local control and the elimination of micrometastases. Effective combination therapy utilizing surgery and radiotherapy has improved the functional outcome without compromising local control of the primary tumor, particularly in soft tissue sarcomas of the extremities. Metastases, however, occur in up to half of the cases, even with adequate local control [1-3]. This chapter will update studies reviewed in the last volume of this series and discuss new relevant information and topics.

Published clinical trials in soft tissue sarcoma are difficult to evaluate and compare. These tumors are rare, and few studies have accrued more than 100 patients. In addition, histologic classification is difficult, and the interaction of a number of pathologic subtypes, histologic grades, and primary tumor locations may result in imbalances of prognostic factors between randomized groups, particularly within the smaller trials, which may not be entirely compensated for by stratification or Cox regression analysis.

Randomized Trials of Adjuvant Chemotherapy

This chapter concentrates on a review of randomized studies of adjuvant chemotherapy, which include a concurrent control group. General criteria of eligibility for many of these studies have been detailed in Volume 2.

Doxorubicin vs. Control

Table 1 summarizes the results of five trials, each of which examines the outcome of a group receiving adjuvant doxorubicin (DX) in comparison

Pinedo, H.M., Verweij, J., and H.D. Suit (eds.): Soft Tissue Sarcomas: New Developments in the Multidisciplinary Approach to Treatment. © *1991 Kluwer Academic Publishers, Boston. ISBN: 0–7923–1139–6. All rights reserved.*

Table 1. Adjuvant chemotherapy: Randomized studies of doxorubicin vs. control.

Center	Treatment	No. evaluable patients	Median FU months	LR[c]	Mets.[c]	RFS (%)[c]	OS (%)[c]
Boston/ECOG[b] [4] (1978—1985)	DX[a]	37	} 49 } (16—80)	3	NS[e]	74 } $p = 0.11$	68 } $p = 0.23$
	Control	38		4	NS	62	68
UCLA[c] [6] (1981—1984)	DX	56	28	2[f]	NS	58 } n.s.	85 } n.s.[c]
	Control	63		7[f]	NS	54	80
Intergroup[b] (USA) [7] (1983—1987)	DX	32	} 20 } (1—39)	NS	NS	67 } n.s.	82 } n.s.
	Control	32		NS	NS	67	89
Scandinavia[b,g] [10] (1981—1986)	DX	77	40	NS	NS	62 } n.s.	75 } NS
	Control	77		NS	NS	56	70
Bologna[c] [11,12] (1981→)	DX	33	36[d]	4	7	68 } $p < 0.02$	88 } $p < 0.05$
	Control	44		7	22	42	68

[a] DX = doxorubicin.
[b] Sarcomas, all sites.
[c] Extremity sarcomas only.
[d] Approximate; actual value not stated.
[e] FU = follow-up; LR = local recurrence; Mets. = metastases; n.s. = not significant; NS = not stated; OS = overall survival; and RFS = relapse-free survival.
[f] LR alone. Six patients had simultaneous LR plus mets.
[g] Patients with marginal resection plus postoperative radiotherapy excluded.

with a randomized control group treated only by surgery with or without radiotherapy.

Boston/ECOG [4]   As reported in Volume 3, no significant differences were found between the treatment arm (in which patients received DX 90 mg/m² every 3 weeks for 5 courses) and the control arm, with respect to local control, metastasis-free survival, relapse-free survival (RFS), and overall survival (OS). Subgroup analysis failed to show evidence of a benefit from DX therapy for either extremity or for nonextremity sarcomas.

UCLA [5,6]   As previously described, a group of patients with extremity soft tissue sarcoma, all receiving preoperative intra-arterial DX (20 to 30 mg/day continuously for 3 days) and preoperative irradiation on protocol, were also entered into a prospective randomized study of adjuvant DX (45 mg/m² daily × 2, every 4 weeks for 5 courses), starting within 6 weeks of surgery, vs. control. A full paper on this study [6], with median follow-up of 28 months, confirmed an earlier abstract report [5] that had found no significant differences in terms of local recurrence, RFS, or OS. There was a slightly lower local recurrence rate in those patients who received adjuvant systemic DX, but this did not reach statistical significance. The infusion of DX intra-arterially to both groups may have obscured any difference between the arms.

Intergroup (USA) [7,8]   A preliminary analysis of this trial was published in abstract form [7], and a brief report appeared in a symposium proceedings [8]. However, the latter presented little new information. Patients were randomized to DX 70 mg/m², with escalation to 90 mg/m² every 3 weeks for a total of 6 courses. Although 114 patients were randomized, the symposium report updates the initial 81 patients, and median follow-up is not stated. In the extremity subgroup (41 patients), a trend toward improved RFS for the DX group was noted ($p = 0.06$), but OS was not significantly different.

Scandinavian Sarcoma Group [9,10]   A full report of this study, the largest using adjuvant DX, has now been published. Over 5 years, 240 patients with high-grade (Broder's III and IV) sarcomas were randomized to receive DX 60 mg/m² monthly for 9 courses, or no systemic treatment. Sixty-nine patients (29%) were not evaluable, with the most common reasons for exclusion being ineligible histologies (22 patients) or marginal excisions not followed by radiotherapy (25 patients). Thirty-four patients who underwent a marginal resection received radiotherapy postoperatively before being randomized and were analyzed separately. No patients were lost to follow-up, and median follow-up was 40 months. No significant differences between the treatment and the control groups were seen with respect to local recurrence, RFS, or OS, either for the 181 evaluable or the 240 total randomized patients. The authors concluded that "...the use of single-agent doxorubicin as postoperative adjuvant chemotherapy has no significant clinical benefit in patients with high-grade soft tissue sarcoma."

Bologna [11,12]   This study, last updated in 1987, remains the only study that supports the use of adjuvant single-agent DX. The surgical groups and treatment regimens were detailed in Volume 3. Particular criticisms of this study, as outlined in the previous volume, are a large imbalance in patient numbers between treatment groups, and a possible excess of poor prognosis (thigh/buttock) tumors in the control group, which may account for an unexpectedly poor RFS figure for the control group.

Combination Chemotherapy

Table 2 summarizes the results of randomized studies evaluating combination chemotherapy.

M.D. Anderson [13]   This study was updated in 1987 after 10 years of follow-up and was reviewed in Volume 3. The first report, with median follow-up of 18 months, found that RFS did not differ significantly between chemotherapy and the control groups. The subsequent report, after 10 yrs of follow-up, revealed that RFS favored the chemotherapy group, although OS was not significantly different. The explanation for this finding was a reduced local recurrence rate in the chemotherapy group. Metastases occurred with similar frequency in the two arms.

Mayo Clinic [14]   Again, no further information has become available since the study was reviewed in Volume 2.

National Cancer Institute [15,16]   This study has been updated [16], with median follow-up of 7.1 years. For extremity sarcomas, RFS was significantly better ($p = 0.04$), while OS, although favoring the chemotherapy arm, was not significantly different ($p = 0.12$). All previous reports have documented a benefit in terms of overall survival. Local recurrences were significantly decreased ($p = <0.05$) in the chemotherapy arm. This study, like the Bologna study, suffers from an imbalance in numbers between the randomized groups, and the total accrual (67 pts) was small. The study of nonextremity sarcomas has not been updated and was reviewed in Volume 2.

  A second trial compared the original high-dose DX chemotherapy with a second regimen utilizing lower doses of DX in order to avoid anthracycline-associated cardiomyopathy. Eighty-eight patients were accrued, and 5-year RFS (72%) and OS (75%) were not significantly different between high- and low-dose chemotherapy arms.

Table 2. Adjuvant chemotherapy: Randomized studies of combination chemotherapy vs. control.

Center[b]	Treatment[a]	Site	No. evaluable patients	Median FU months	LR[e]	Mets.[e]	RFS (%)[e]	OS (%)[e]
M.D. Anderson [13] (1973—1976)	VCR-DX-CTX-DACT	Limb	20	>120	2	9	54 } $p = 0.04$	65 } $p = 0.25$
	Control		23		8	11	35	
Mayo Clinic [14] (1975—1981)	VCR-CTX-DACT alternating VCR-DX-DTIC	Limb Abdomen[c]	26 4			NS	NS[e]	90 } $p = 0.55$
	Control	Limb Abdomen[c]	26 5	64	17	NS	NS	77
NCI [15,16] (1977—1981)	DX-CTX-HDMTX	Limb	39	85	1	NS	75 } $p = 0.04$	82 } $p = 0.12$
	Control		28		4	NS	54	60
	DX-CTX-HDMTX	Head,[d] neck, trunk	17	35	NS	NS	77 } $p = 0.08$	68 } $p = 0.38$
	Control		14		NS	NS	49	58
EORTC [18,19] (1978)	CTX-VCR-DX-DTIC	All	178	44	22	NS	67 } $p = 0.01$	74 } $p = 0.26$
	Control		196		44	NS	52	68
Fondation Bergonie [20]	CTX-VCR-DX-DTIC	All	31	40	1	NS	NS	83 } $p = 0.002$
	Control		28		5	NS	NS	43

a CTX = cytoxan (cyclophosphamide); DACT = actinomycin D; DX = doxorubicin; DTIC = dacarbazine; CR = vincristine; HDMTX = high dose methotrexate.
b Mayo Clinic, 25% low grade; NCI, no low grade; EORTC, 18% low grade; and Fondation Bergonie, no low grade.
c Includes retroperitoneal.
d Excludes retroperitoneal.
e LR = local recurrence; Mets. = metastases; NS = not stated; OS = overall survival; RFS = relapse-free survival; and FU = follow-up.

EORTC [17-19]   This study, which accrued patients from 1977 to 1988, is now complete and has been updated in abstract form [19]. It remains the largest trial of adjuvant chemotherapy in soft tissue sarcomas, with 468 patients randomized to either CYVADIC (cyclophosphamide, vincristine, DX, and dacarbazine) given over 3 days every 4 weeks for 8 courses, beginning within 13 weeks of definitive surgery, or no treatment. There were 374 patients eligible, with a median follow-up time of 44 months. Local recurrence was significantly reduced in the chemotherapy arm ($p = 0.004$), but this finding was confined to the nonextremity sarcomas ($p = 0.003$), with no difference for limb tumors ($p = 0.38$). There were no significant differences in time to distance metastases, or survival. The size of the primary tumor ($p = 0.03$) and histological grade were independent prognostic factors for survival.

Fondation Bergonie, France [20]   The first report of this trial has appeared in abstract form. Fifty-nine patients were randomized to receive 8 to 11 courses of CYVADIC every 3 weeks, commencing within 4 weeks of surgery. There were 36 extremity and 23 nonextremity (no visceral) tumors grouped as 11 cases, stage IIb; 37 cases, stage III; and 11 cases, steps IVa. Median follow-up was 40 months. A trend ($p = 0.17$) towards improvement in the local recurrence rate was seen in the chemotherapy group. In contrast, a significant difference in 5-year metastasis-free survival (65% vs. 34%; $p = 0.003$) and 5-year OS (83% vs. 43%; $p = 0.002$) favoring the chemotherapy group was seen. Prognostic factor analysis suggested maximum benefit of chemotherapy for grade 3 as well as for deep-seated and large tumors and those located in an extremity.

Comment

It is intriguing to note that an increasing number of studies, particularly those using combination chemotherapy, find that this treatment is associated with a reduction in LR, although most do not demonstrate a concomitant reduction in metastases or improvement in overall survival. Significant differences in LR between chemotherapy and control arms have been demonstrated in the M.D. Anderson, NCI, and EORTC trials, and a similar trend is noted in the Fondation Bergonie study. The only study of combination chemotherapy that does not show this effect (Mayo Clinic) omitted local radiotherapy and gave inadequate chemotherapy. The effect is less clear for adjuvant single-agent DX. Although the UCLA and Bologna studies show small decreases in LR following chemotherapy, no such effect is evident in the Boston/ECOG and Scandinavian studies, and insufficient information is available for the Intergroup trial.

As noted in Volume 3, the only studies that have shown significant differences in RFS and OS (Bologna and NCI) have been criticized on statistical grounds. The recent abstract from Fondation Bergonie is interesting. Like the EORTC trial, CYVADIC was the adjuvant chemotherapy regimen, although the doses and schedule used at the Fondation are not stated. Only 46% of patients in the EORTC trial received radiotherapy compared with 93% in the French study. Also, not stated in the Fondation trial is the proportion of patients with microscopic residual disease. The Fondation study is considerably smaller than the EORTC trial and may be more subject to imbalances between the treatment arms. On the other hand, CYVADIC was started within 4 weeks of surgery in the Fondation trial compared with 13 weeks in the EORTC trial. The shortened time to treatment may enhance the effect of chemotherapy. A detailed comparison of these trials awaits definitive publications of each.

Quality of Life Issues

In the adjuvant situation, benefits in terms of freedom from local or distant recurrence and overall survival have to be balanced against short- and long-term toxicities. In all areas of oncology, increasing attention is being paid to these quality-of-life issues, and the management of soft tissue sarcomas is no exception. The major areas of interest have revolved about the benefits (often presumed) of limb-salvage procedures (see Chapter 5) and long-term adverse side effects of chemotherapy, including gonadal function.

Doxorubicin-Induced Cardiomyopathy

As noted in Volume 3, the NCI group reported a high incidence of DX-associated cardiomyopathy in patients treated with the original combination chemotherapy regimen [15]. There were 101 patients prospectively assessed [21], of which 75 underwent one or more radionuclide angiogram (RNA) to document left ventricular ejection fraction. Fourteen developed congestive heart failure, but in the asymptomatic group, 52% of RNA were abnormal. The same investigators went on to assess prospectively 118 patients with soft tissue sarcoma treated on various NCI protocols [22]. Sixty-two patients recieved high-dose DX (50 mg/m^2/month increased by 10 mg/m^2 to a maximum of 70 mg/m^2) with cyclophosphamide and high-dose methotrexate, achieving a planned cumulative DX dose of 530 mg/m^2. Fifty-six patients received low-dose doxorubicin (70 mg/m^2/month) with cyclophosphamide, reaching a planned cumulative DX dose of 350 mg/m^2. Although doses were adjusted for myelosuppression, the actual cumulative doses of DX for high- and low-dose groups were 452 ± 156 mg/m^2 and 319 ± 77 mg/m^2, respectively. Symptomatic congestive heart failure was not seen in this study, in contrast with the first series, but declines in left ventricular ejection fraction were seen in both groups; a greater number of

RNA values changed from normal to abnormal (22 vs. 11) in the high-dose DX group, although the difference was not statistically significant.

Gonadal Function

The NCI group examined 11 women aged 16 to 43 [23] and 26 men aged 16 to 63 [24] who received adjuvant chemotherapy (doxorubicin, cyclophosphamide, and high-dose methotrexate) with or without radiotherapy for soft tissue sarcoma. None of the patients had a history of abnormal development, infertility, or irregular menses before treatment, and none of the women were maintained on oral contraceptives after treatment. Luteinizing hormone (LH), follicle stimulating hormone (FSH), and the appropriate target hormone levels (testosterone or estradiol) were measured as well as testicular size. Monthly semen analyses were performed, and a menstrual history was taken.

Five women received chemotherapy alone, and the three younger women (16, 17, and 32 years) developed minimal menstrual irregularities or temporary cessation of menses while on treatment, but with return to normal periods after treatment had ended. The two older women in the group (36 and 42 years) had persistent irregular or absent menses, with marked elevation of FSH levels and depressed estradiol concentrations. Four women received chemotherapy and radiotherapy "distal" to the ovaries (chest, leg, or thigh). Similarly, the two younger women (16 and 23 years) had a return of normal menstrual function at the end of the treatment, but the two older women (38 and 43 years) had persistent absence of menses or extremely infrequent menses associated with elevated gonadotropin and reduced estradiol levels. Only two women received chemotherapy and pelvic irradiation (7,000 cGy). Both had castrate levels of all three measured hormones.

Six men received chemotherapy alone. Three of five men for whom semen analyses were available had normal sperm counts and plasma hormone concentrations. One man remained oligospermic, and one remained azoospermic, both having elevated FSH levels, with testosterone and LH levels indistinguishable from normal. Eleven patients received chemotherapy and "distal radiotherapy" (arm, neck, chest, or lower leg). Sperm counts were available on eight patients, of whom two had normal sperm concentrations, three were oligospermic, and three were azoospermic. Testosterone levels were similar to those of normal men. Nine patients received chemotherapy and "proximal radiotherapy" (thigh, abdomen, or pelvis). Eight men had ejaculates analyzed, and all were azoospermic and had elevated levels of gonadotropin, but normal testosterone. These patients remain azoospermic 2 to 3 years after treatment, whereas some men who received "distal" or no radiotherapy, recovered normal testicular function. The authors suggest that recovery is more likely at ages 40 years or less.

Continuing Research in Adjuvant Chemotherapy

The poor prognosis of many patients with resectable soft tissue sarcomas, the equivocal results obtained thus far in randomized clinical trials, and the introduction of new agents and combinations continue to spur cooperative oncology group efforts in this area. An Intergroup trial, utilizing the combination of DX, dacarbazine, and ifosfamide with the uroprotectant Mesna, compared to no treatment, is currently underway. Four different types of local control procedures (radical resection with or without postoperative radiotherapy; preoperative external beam irradiation followed by surgery followed by postoperative external beam irradiation boost; surgery [wide excision] followed by postoperative external beam irradiation; the Eilber technique of intra-arterial DX plus preoperative external beam irradiation followed by surgery) are permitted in this trial. The NCI Group is currently randomizing patients with extremity soft tissue sarcoma, who have received surgery and adjuvant chemotherapy with cyclophosphamide (700 mg/m^2) and doxorubicin (70 mg/m^2) monthly for five courses, to postoperative radiotherapy or no further treatment. The radiotherapy in the treatment arm will begin within 2 to 3 days of the commencement of chemotherapy. The aims of this study are to evaluate the combined toxicities of chemotherapy and irradiation and to assess differences in rates of local control. For patients who have tumors arising in the head and neck regions, breast, or trunk, all patients will be treated by surgery and radiotherapy and then randomized to the combination of cyclophosphamide and DX, or no chemotherapy.

An EORTC study that opened in June 1988 evaluates neoadjuvant chemotherapy in patients with poor prognosis soft tissue sarcomas of the extremities, head, neck, and trunk. Three courses of chemotherapy with DX, ifosfamide, and Mesna are administered before definitive surgery and radiotherapy. There are four stratification groups: (1) tumor >8 cm, any histological grade; (2) tumor ≤8 cm, grades II and III only; (3) inadequately resected tumor requiring further surgery, grades II and III; and (4) local recurrence, grades II and III. Chemotherapy must commence within 6 weeks of biopsy or an attempt at definitive surgery.

The results of these trials will help to define the appropriate place for adjuvant chemotherapy in the management of these diseases.

References

1. Suit HD: Patterns of failure after treatment of sarcoma of soft tissue by radical surgery or by conservative surgery and radiation. Cancer Treat Symp 2:241—246, 1983.
2. Potter DA, Glenn J, Kinsella T, Glatstein E, Lack EE, Restrepo C, White DE, Seipp CA, Wesley R, Rosenberg SA: Patterns of recurrence in patients with high-grade soft tissue sarcomas. J Clin Oncol 3:353—366, 1985.

3. Romsdahl MM, Lindberg RD, Martin RG: Patterns of failure after treatment of soft tissue sarcoma. Cancer Treat Symp 2:251—258, 1983.
4. Wilson RE, Wood WC, Lerner HL, Antman K, Amato D, Corson JM, Proppe K, Harmon D, Carey R, Greenberger J, Suit H: Doxorubicin chemotherapy in the treatment of soft tissue sarcoma: Combined results of two randomized trials. Arch Surg 121:1354—1359, 1986.
5. Eilber FR, Ciuliano AE, Huth JF, Morton DL: Adjuvant adriamycin in high-grade extremity soft tissue sarcoma: A randomized prospective trial. Proc Am Soc Clin Oncol 5:125, 1986.
6. Eilber FR, Giuliano AE, Huth JF, Morton DL: A randomized prospective trial using postoperative adjuvant chemotherapy (adriamycin) in high-grade extremity soft tissue sarcoma. Amer J Clin Oncol (CCT) 11:39—45, 1988.
7. Antman K, Amato D, Pilepich M, et al.: Preliminary results of a randomized Intergroup soft tissue sarcoma adjuvant trial of doxorubicin versus observation. In: Adjuvant therapy of cancer. Salmon VS (ed). Philadelphia: Grune and Stratton, p 725, 1987.
8. Baker LH: Adjuvant therapy for soft tissue sarcomas. In: Recent concepts in sarcoma treatment. Ryan JR, Baker LO (eds). Dordrecht, The Netherlands: Kluwer Academic Publishers, pp 131—136, 1988.
9. Alvegard TA: Adjuvant chemotherapy with adriamycin in high grade malignant soft tissue sarcoma: A Scandinavian randomized study. Proc Am Soc Clin Oncol 5:125, 1986.
10. Alvegard RA, Sigurdson H, Mouridsen H, Soiheim O, Unsgaard D, Ringborg U, Dahl O, Nordentoft AM, Blomqvist C, Rydholm A, Stener B, Ranstam J: Adjuvant chemotherapy with doxorubicin in high-grade soft tissue sarcoma: A randomized trial of the Scandinavian Sarcoma Group. J Clin Oncol 7:1504—1513, 1989.
11. Gherlinzoni F, Bacci G, Picci P, Lapanna R, Calderoni P, Lorenzi EG, Bernini M, Emiliani E, Barbieri E, Mormand A, Campanacci M: A randomized trial for the treatment of high grade soft tissue sarcomas of the extremities: Preliminary observations. J Clin Oncol 4:552—558, 1986.
12. Picci P, Bacci G, Gherlinzoni F, Capanna R, Mercuri M, Ruggieri P, Baldini N, Avella M, Pignatti G, Manfrini M: Results of a randomized trial for the treatment of localized soft tissue tumors (STS) of the extremities in adult patients. In: Recent concepts in sarcoma treatment. Ryan JR, Baker LO (eds). Dordrecht, The Netherlands: Kluwer Academic Publishers, pp 144—148, 1988.
13. Benjamin RS, Terjanian TO, Genoglio CJ, Barkley HT, Evans HC, Murphy WK, Martin RG: The importance of combination chemotherapy for adjuvant treatment of high risk patients with soft tissue sarcomas of the extremities. In: Adjuvant therapy of cancer V. New York: Grune and Stratton, pp 735—744, 1987.
14. Edmonson JH, Fleming TR, Ivins VC, Burgert EO, Souie EH, O'Connell MJ, Sim FH, Ahmann DL: Randomized study of systemic chemotherapy following complete excision of non-osseous sarcomas. J Clin Oncol 2:1390—1396, 1984.
15. Baker AR, Change AE, Glatstein E, Rosenberg SA: National Cancer Institute experience in the management of high grade extremity soft tissue sarcoma. In: Recent concepts in sarcoma treatment. Dordrecht, The Netherlands: Kluwer Academic Publishers, pp 123—130, 1988.
16. Chang AR, Kinsella R, Glatstein E, Baker AR, Sindecar WF, Lotze MT, Danforth DN, Sugarbaker PH, Lack EE, Steinberg SM, White DE, Rosenberg SA: Adjuvant chemotherapy for patients with high grade soft tissue sarcomas of the extremity. J Clin Oncol 6:1491—1500, 1988.
17. Bramwell VHC, Rouesse J, Santoro A, Buesa J, Somers R, Thomas D, Sylvester R, Pinedo HM: European experience of adjuvant chemotherapy for soft tissue sarcomas: Preliminary report of a randomized trial of cyclophosphamide, vincristine, doxorubicin and dacarbazine. Cancer Treat Symp 3:99—108, 1985.
18. Bramwell VHC, Rouesse J, Steward W, Santoro A, Buesa J, Schafford–Koops N, Wagener T, Somers R, Ruka W, Markham D, Burgers M, Van Unnik J, Comtesso G, Thomas D,

102

Sylvester R, Pinedo H: European experience of adjuvant chemotherapy for soft tissue sarcoma: An interim report of a randomized trial of CYVADIC versus control. In: Recent concepts in sarcoma treatment. Dordrecht, The Netherlands: Kluwer Academic Publishers, pp 157—164, 1988.

19. Bramwell V, Rouesse J, Steward W, Santoro A, Buesa J, Thomas D, Sylvester R: Reduced rate of local recurrence following CYVADIC chemotherapy in localized soft tissue sarcoma: An EORTC randomized trial. Proc Am Soc Clin Oncol 8:320, 1989.

20. Bui NB, Maree D, Coindre JM, Bonichon F, Kantor G, Avril A, Ravaud A: First results of a prospective randomized study of CYVADIC adjuvant chemotherapy in adults with operable high risk soft tissue sarcoma. Proc Am Soc Clin Oncol 8:318, 1989.

21. Dresdale A, Bonow RO, Wesley R, Palmeri ST, Barr L, Mathison D, D'Abngelo T, Rosenberg SA: Prospective evaluation of doxorubicin-induced cardiomyopathy resulting from postsurgical adjuvant treatment of patients with soft tissue sarcomas. Cancer 52:51—60, 1983.

22. Ettinghausen SE, Bonow RO, Palmeri ST, Seipp CA, Steinberg SM, White DE, Rosenberg SA: Prospective study of cardiomyopathy induced by adjuvant doxorubicin therapy in patients with soft tissue sarcomas. Arch Surg 121:1445—1451, 1986.

23. Shamberger RC, Sherins RJ, Ziegler JL, Glatstein E, Rosenberg SA: Effects of postoperative adjuvant chemotherapy and radiotherapy on ovarian function in women undergoing treatment for soft tissue sarcoma. J Natl Cancer Inst 67:1213—1218, 1981.

24. Shamberger RC, Sherins RJ, Rosenberg SA: The effects of postoperative adjuvant chemotherapy and radiotherapy in testicular function in men undergoing treatment for soft tissue sarcoma. Cancer 47:2368—2374, 1981.

9. Pre- and Perioperative Perfusion Chemotherapy for Soft Tissue Sarcoma of the Limbs

Michael Meyer, James H. Muchmore, and Edward T. Krementz

Introduction

Soft tissue sarcomas are relatively rare tumors. Each year in the U.S., there are approximately 5,500 new cases and 2,900 deaths attributed to these tumors [1,2]. Approximately 60% of these tumors develop in the extremities.

Surgical therapy characteristically has been associated with high local recurrence rates, varying from more than 90% with local excision, 20 to 40% with wide radical resection, to 7 to 18% following amputation [3-8].

Since the advent of regional chemotherapy techniques in the 1950s by Klopp et al. [9] and Bierman et al. [10], radical surgical therapy has gradually given way to multimodal treatment plans involving preoperative regional chemotherapy with and without radiation therapy, allowing a more conservative surgical resection and resulting in better limb preservation. Preoperative regional chemotherapy may be given by intra-arterial infusion or perioperative chemotherapy by regional perfusion, a technique developed in 1957 by Creech, Krementz, and Ryan at the Tulane University School of Medicine [11,12]. The perfusion technique has been instrumental in helping to define the capabilities of regional chemotherapy and has permitted about a 90% limb-salvage rate in patients with soft tissue sarcoma of the extremities [13,14].

This chapter will review our experience with preoperative intra-arterial chemotherapy and those reported in the literature. We will also review the Tulane experience with perioperative regional chemotherapy administered by isolated regional perfusion, and the accomplishments of others using this modality.

Preoperative Chemotherapy by Intra-arterial Infusion

The direct arterial administration of regional chemotherapy by infusion, although lacking the multiple advantages of isolation, is in some aspects more versatile than perfusion, since it can be used for any anatomically

Pinedo, H.M., Verweij, J., and H.D. Suit (eds.): Soft Tissue Sarcomas: New Developments in the Multidisciplinary Approach to Treatment. © *1991 Kluwer Academic Publishers, Boston. ISBN: 0-7923-1139-6. All rights reserved.*

confined regional tumor. Regional intra-arterial chemotherapy has been used for tumors of the breast [15,16], head and neck [17], liver [18-20], pelvis [21,22], and limbs [23-29]. Treatment schedules can be adapted to include a wider variety of chemotherapeutic agents, including the antimetabolites, which are much more effective when administered over long time periods as compared to short-term perfusions more suitable for rapidly acting agents. Also, therapy can be administered on an outpatient basis and repeated periodically on multiple occasions. Since the introduction of arterial drug administration in the 1950s, better techniques for the safe percutaneous introduction of infusion catheters under fluoroscopy have greatly expanded the use of intra-arterial chemotherapy. In addition, the use of implantable catheters has all but eliminated the primary complications of bleeding, catheter displacement, and infection. The development of permanent or semipermanent implantable intra-arterial ports has been a great advantage to the administration of fractional or continuous regional chemotherapy. The well-tolerated sialastic tubing now available in small diameters can be used in tributary arteries, and the newer ports with large access windows that tolerate innumerable needle sticks continue to make this technique more attractive for use. Figure 1 shows examples of the placement of intra-arterial catheters in access vessels used for chemotherapy of head and neck tumors, upper limb or axillary tumors, or inguinal or lower limb tumors.

The principle advantage of chemotherapy administered intra-arterially is an augmentation of both the regional plasma peak concentration of the agent and the area under the concentration-time curve (AUC) [30]. This has been demonstrated clinically for a number of chemotherapeutic agents, such as 5-fluorouracil [31], cisplatin [32], doxorubicin [33], carmustine [31], streptozocin [34], and mitomycin-C [31]. Increased local tissue concentrations of drugs following intra-arterial administration have also been documented for cisplatin [35], carmustine [36], doxorubicin [37], methotrexate (MTX) [38], bleomycin [39], and etoposide [40]. This increase in regional plasma and tissue drug concentrations can potentially translate into augmentation of local antitumor efficacy, since most chemotherapeutic agents have a relatively steep dose-response curve [30,31].

Local toxicity does occur with intra-arterial administration of a drug, occasionally producing severe local skin toxicity [16] and/or peripheral neuropathies [21]. Vesicants, such as doxorubicin, when administered by rapid arterial infusion, are poorly tolerated and should be given by prolonged infusion. Extravasation of drugs such as doxorubicin may cause necrosis and sloughing of surrounding tissues. These drugs can also produce local arteritis. Other infrequent complications include vascular trauma secondary to catheter placement (including intimal dissections), thrombosis, and stenosis [41]. Infections developing in an implanted port or arterial line can cause serious recurring problems and are best handled by removal of the port and catheter.

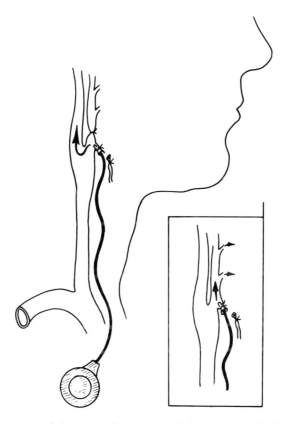

Figure 1A. Access routes and placement of permanent subcutaneous ports for long term administration of intra-arterial regional chemotherapy. Ports and catheter usually placed under local anesthesia. Distribution flow is monitored with Fluorocite© and Wood's light or with indigo carmine or other vital dyes. (Figure 1A.) Access route for brain and/or ophthalmic artery (first branch of internal carotid) for orbital or ocular neoplasms. For oropharyngeal lesions supplied by external carotid artery (see insert), the external carotid is left patent. Catheter introduced through the superior thyroid artery. External carotid artery is ligated if flow is to be directed into internal carotid. Port is placed over second thoracic interspace.

Eilber et al. [23], expanding on the early experience of regional chemotherapy, designed a preoperative treatment strategy using both regional intra-arterial doxorubicin and rapid-fraction irradiation as adjunctive treatment with the purpose of achieving better local disease control and limb salvage in patients who would otherwise require amputation. Doxorubicin, introduced in the 1970s, remains one of the most effective single agents for the treatment of sarcoma, although current experience with cisplatin indicates that this agent has great potential for intermittent intra-arterial use for sarcoma, particularly when combined with hyperthermia. Regional infusions of doxorubicin may increase its tissue concentration because it is not diluted, and the drug fixes avidly to local tissues. Moreover, doxorubicin

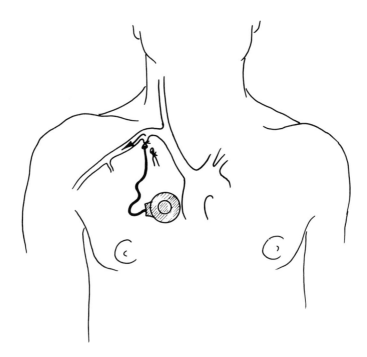

Figure 1B. Access for axillary or upper limb tumors. Sialastic catheter inserted through thoraco-acromial or long thoracic artery. Port is placed over medial aspect of second thoracic interspace.

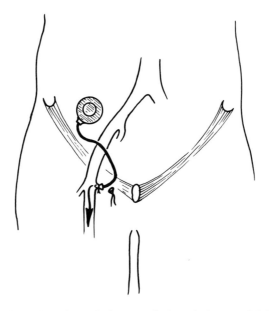

Figure 1C. Access for groin or lower limb tumors is through the superficial epigastric artery or superficial circumflex artery. Port is placed over lower abdomen or upper thigh.

is thought to be a radiation sensitizer, since it enhances the effect of ionizing radiation.

Eilber reported on three sequential treatment programs [23]. A group of 55 patients received "standard" therapy, which included amputation (19 patients), wide excision (11 patients), or wide excision followed by 5,000 to 6,000 cGy of radiation (25 patients). The local recurrence rate in this group was 25%. A second group of 77 patients received intra-arterial doxorubicin, 30 mg/day for 3 days, followed by radiation therapy of 350 cGy for 10 days (3,500 cGy). The limb-salvage rate was 96%, and the local recurrence rate fell to 4%. However, the complication rate was 35%, including wound sloughing (19%) and pathologic fractures of long bones (8%). Because of the high complication rate, the treatment program was altered to reduce the radiation dose by one half, from 3,600 to 1,750 cGy. Of the 105 patients treated, the limb-salvage rate remained a good 97%; however, the local recurrence rate doubled to 8%. The complication rate decreased to 25%, including wound slough (16%) and pathologic fracture of long bones (<1%). The survival rate in this group of patients, after a median follow-up of 24 months, was 95%. This compared with a survival rate of 64% after a median follow-up of 5 years in the group receiving 3,500 cGy.

Mantravadi et al. [24] treated 32 patients having high-grade soft tissue sarcomas of the extremity, with preoperative intra-arterial infusion of doxorubicin (10 mg/M^2 day for 10 days) followed by radiation therapy of 250 cGy/day for 10 days. En bloc resection was then performed. Post-operatively, depending upon the surgical specimen findings, radiation therapy was given to a dose ranging from 5,000 cGy in 5 weeks to 6,000 cGy in 6 weeks. No residual tumor was found in 28% of the surgical specimens, and only minimal tumor in 41%. A functionally intact limb was preserved in 30 patients (94%). Local recurrence developed in only one patient (3%). The actuarial overall survival at 3 years was 70%, and disease-free survival 57%.

Denton et al. [25] treated 20 patients having soft tissue sarcoma and ten patients having skeletal sarcomas, with intra-arterial doxorubicin (100 mg over 3 days), followed within 10 days by rapid-fraction irradiation (3,000 cGy or 300 cGy fractions × ten, over a 2-week period) prior to surgical excision of the tumor. Most patients had large high-grade tumors. The size and location of the sarcoma permitted only a marginal resection in one half of the patients, while the remainder could be excised in a three-dimensional en bloc manner. Most patients received postoperative systemic doxorubicin chemotherapy (450 mg/M^2 total dose given intravenously over 6 months). Two of six patients with significant wound complications later required amputation. Only one patient developed a local recurrence after a mean follow-up of 22 months, and 85% of the patients had a functional extremity. The 3-year survival rate was 68% for soft tissue sarcoma. Three patients subsequently required amputation, resulting in an overall limb salvage rate of 90%.

Goodnight et al. [26] treated 17 patients having soft tissue sarcoma of the limb, with preoperative intra-arterial doxorubicin followed by rapid-fraction radiation therapy. Functional limbs were salvaged in 15 patients, with no local recurrence. Overall survival after a median follow-up of 32 months was 82%, and disease-free survival was 59%. Five patients (29%) required a second procedure for closure. Two patients had pathologic fractures of underlying long bones (one femur and one humerus) 12 and 25 months after treatment. The authors note that the stripping of periosteum from the radiated underlying long bone to achieve a tumor-free margin may predispose to pathologic fracture.

Stephens et al. [27] reported the use of combined intra-arterial doxorubicin and cisplatin as the initial treatment before subsequent radiotherapy and/or surgery in the treatment of three locally advanced osteogenic sarcomas and five locally advanced soft tissue sarcomas in the shoulder, pelvis, and thigh. In each case, the tumor regressed in size after several courses of chemotherapy, and needle biopsies of tumor to confirm tumor response revealed no evidence of residual sarcoma in five patients (63%). Seven patients had surgical resection of the residual tumor mass after three to six courses of chemotherapy, and apparently viable tumor cells were found in four of the resected specimens (57%). Residual tumor cells were found in one of three patients with soft tissue sarcomas given postinfusion radiotherapy before surgery. Four patients developed lung metastases after treatment. Four patients remained well with no local recurrence or metastatic disease developing between 1 to 3.5 years after presentation. Limb salvage was possible in seven patients.

Hoekstra et al. [28] have treated nine patients having a high-grade soft tissue sarcoma of an extremity, with preoperative intra-arterial doxorubicin and postoperative radiotherapy and conservative surgical resection. Limb salvage was possible in eight patients. During a median follow-up of 24 months, one local recurrence and four distant metastases were diagnosed. Four patients developed complications due to the intra-arterial chemotherapy. Patients with demonstrable tumor destruction after the combined therapy had a longer disease-free survival.

Azzarelli et al. [29] used 8 days of continuous doxorubicin infusion for two preoperative cycles (100 mg/M^2 per cycle) in the treatment of limb soft tissue sarcomas. They also found a significantly better survival in patients whose tumors showed a distinct response (more than 75% tumor necrosis) to the chemotherapy.

The Tulane experience with regional intra-arterial chemotherapy in the treatment of 33 patients with soft tissue sarcoma, most of whom had unresectable or advanced disease, was last reported in 1985 [42]. There were 15 with lower limb sarcomas, 4 with upper limb sarcomas, 5 with head and neck tumors, and 9 with lesions of the pelvis, hip, or buttocks. In six cases, chemotherapy was given preoperatively, and in one case, postoperatively as adjuvant therapy. The remaining 26 patients had palliative chemotherapy.

Several rewarding responses of preoperative chemotherapy cases occurred in patients with malignant fibrous histocytomas (MFH) of the hip and buttock. One woman with a large MFH of the buttock was treated with intra-arterial doxorubicin delivered at the common iliac artery and through a retrograde infusion catheter placed in the common femoral artery. The drug was administered fractionally over 6 days. The patient received two additional courses of intravenous doxorubicin. the tumor was reduced insufficiently to permit wide excision after a 6-week interval. Good palliation was achieved, but the patient died of pulmonary metastases approximately 30 months later. Another interesting patient was a 61-year-old man who presented in October 1979 with MFH arising in the area of the soft tissues adjacent to the left ischial tuberosity (approximately 11 × 10 cm in diameter and fixed to the underlying bony structures of the pelvis). A hindquarter resection had been recommended and would have been required for a definitive surgical excision. As the prospect of a major amputation was unacceptable to the patient, he was referred to us for perfusion chemotherapy. The patient received a 5-day course of doxorubicin, receiving 30 mg through the common iliac artery over a 4-hour period daily. The heparin in the arterial infusion catheter was cleared by a flush with normal saline prior to each treatment. The tumor decreased in size and became more mobile. The patient received three more courses of intravenous doxorubicin (80 mg/day) every 4 to 5 weeks. In January 1980 the patient's tumor had decreased by half, and a wide excision of residual tumor was carried out. The patient received two postoperative courses of i.v. doxorubicin. The patient has made a full recovery and remains free of disease 10 years later. One patient with MFH of the thigh and another with rhabdomyosarcoma (RMS) of the shoulder were treated in a similar fashion, resulting in no recurrence of disease locally, but each died of pulmonary metastasis at 12 and 17 months, respectively.

Perioperative Chemotherapy by Regional Perfusion

Chemotherapy by regional perfusion was developed at Tulane University School of Medicine in 1957 and has proved to be an effective method for the treatment of limb melanoma [11,12]. It also has proved to be very useful in the treatment of soft tissue sarcoma of the limb, especially when combined with excisional surgery [13,14]. By isolating the limb by occlusion and canalization of the distal major vessels and a tourniquet to occlude the superficial vessels, high-dose chemotherapy is introduced and continuously perfused throughout the limb (figure 2). The hyperoxygenated perfusate produces a tissue pO_2 of approximately 400 mm of Hg, and the chemotherapy perfusion is maintained by an extracorporeal pump system for about 1 hour. In 1960 the observations of Cavaliere and Giovanella [43] (see Chapter 10) in Rome showed that hyperthermia by perfusion alone would produce major sarcoma remissions. Also, the reports by Stehlin [44] confirmed

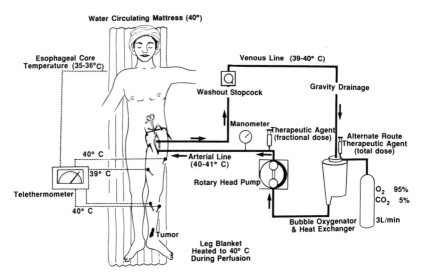

Figure 2. Flow diagram for hyperthermic limb perfusion. Patient is placed on controlled temperature mattress. Under general anesthesia, major limb vessels are exposed; the patient is heparinized and catheterized. Catheters are connected to oxygenator-heat exchanger. Limb is isolated with a tourniquet, and deep subcutaneous thermistor probes are placed in leg and thigh to monitor temperatures. Limb is wrapped with a heating blanket. After desired limb temperatures are achieved, drugs are administered into the arterial line or pump reservoir. Perfusion is continued for 1 hour followed by a wash out with Dextran-40 or whole blood. Catheters are withdrawn, and vessels repaired. Protamine is administered, and planned excisional surgery is performed.

that the combination of chemotherapy and hyperthermia produced even better responses, and currently most perfusions with chemotherapy are generally administered at temperatures ranging from 39 to 41°C.

Technique

For upper limb perfusions, the first portion of the axillary artery and vein are used. Lower limb perfusions are carried out through the external iliac vessels for thigh or groin lesions and through the common femoral vessels for lesions that are below the mid-thigh level. With the patient under general anesthesia, the vessels are exposed, the patient is heparinized, and the vascular catheters are inserted and connected to the extracorporeal, oxygenated bypass system. Whole blood diluted with lactated Ringers solution is used, and the perfusion is begun. A tourniquet around the base of the limb is drawn tight, and isolation is checked with fluorescite administered through the arterial line. Limb temperatures are monitored by subcutaneous thermister probes. A water-circulating heating blanket is used to wrap the limb. Perfusate is usually maintained at 41°C with flow rates of 150 to 400 cc per upper limb and from 200 to 600 cc per lower limb. After the limb temperatures of approximately 40°C are achieved, one or more drugs are given in fractionated doses into the arterial line, and perfusion is carried out for 45 to 60 minutes. Following the perfusion, a washout of residual drug and toxic end products is performed with low molecular weight dextran, and the lost volume is replaced with whole blood. The catheters are withdrawn, vessels repaired, protamine is administered, and surgical procedures are performed as indicated.

Advantages

The rationale for hyperthermic perfusion is extensively reported in Chapter 10. A number of advantages can be derived from the use of regional chemotherapy by perfusion, which are detailed and referenced in other articles [12,46]. They include (1) a six- to tenfold increase in drug concentration over systemic administration can be achieved within the isolated limb; (2) maintenance of an augmented plasma peak concentration during the perfusion of 1 hour maximizes the area under the concentration-time curve (AUC); (3) hyperthermia produces vasodilation within the vasculature, effecting better drug distribution and increasing the metabolism of the isolated tissues of the tumor and the tumor cell uptake of a drug (plus hyperthermia has a selective tumoricidal effect as well); (4) hyperoxygenation of isolated tissue potentiates the action of alkylating agents and has selective tumoricidal effects; (5) heparin is reported to have a tumoricidal activity and antimetastatic effect; (6) isolation of the area decreases systemic toxicity and protects "host resistance"; then lysis of tumor cells in situ may initiate an autoimmunization process; (7) washout of unbound agent and toxic end products decreases systemic toxicity; and (8) reperfusion injury of the tumor cell mass potentiates the effects of hyperthermia and hyperoxygenation. Probably one of the important aspects of the isolated regional perfusion technique is that as the tumor is made ischemic during the placement of access catheters and the connection to a heart-lung pump, it is theorized that as the tumor is reperfused with a hyperthermic, hyperoxygenated perfusate that will selectively damage the tumor cell membranes, the tumor cells with become more susceptible to the uptake of chemotherapeutic agents and their cytotoxicity [47].

Clinical Material

Summarized in Table 1 are the tumor types and the extent of disease treated for 122 patients with limb sarcoma. Fifteen histologic types of sarcomas were presented. Twelve patients has bony tumors; nine had osteogenic sarcoma; two had parosteal sarcoma; and one had Ewing's sarcoma. Staging was performed according to the Tulane Staging System[13]. Stage I includes patients with only localized disease; Stage II includes patients with local

Table 1. 122 Sarcomas of limbs treated by perfusion by stage and tissue type.

	Stage			
	Localized			
	Primary	Recurrent	Regional	Distant
Fibro-	17	3	9	2
MFH*	4	1	1	—
Lipo	10	4	1	1
Muscular	5	1	2	3
Synovial	8	1	1	1
Vascular	4	—	3	—
Lymphatic	2	—	2	—
Neuro-	1	1	—	2
Cartilaginous	—	1	1	2
Periosteal	2	—	—	—
Osteogenic	7	1	—	1
Ewing's	—	—	—	1
Mesodermal	3	—	—	—
Epitheloid	2	—	1	—
Unclassified	7	1	1	1
Total	72	14	22	14

* Malignant fibrous histiocytoma.

recurrences and extensive regional disease more than 5 cm in diameter and patients with regional soft tissue or nodal metastases. Stage III involved distant metastases. A total of 72 patients had Stage I localized tumors; 56 had perfusion as initial treatment followed by excision, whereas 16 underwent perfusion as the only treatment of their disease. A total of 36 patients had Stage II extensive regional disease or metastases. Eleven of 14 patients with locally recurrent Stage II disease had perfusion and wide excision. There were 14 Stage III patients with distant disease, and perfusion was undertaken mainly to control a bulky, painful, or disabling limb tumor. There were 62 males in the series; 19 presented with upper limb lesions, and 43 with lower limb lesions. Of the 60 female patients, 18 had upper limb lesions, and 42 had lower limb lesions. In the series of 122 cases, 40 patients were Black and 82 were Caucasian. Fourteen patients were under age 20, and 12 were in their 20s. Eighteen patients were over 70; however, the peak incidence consisted of those patients in their sixth decade.

The drugs selected for use were relatively equally divided between three groups; nitrogen mustard (HN$_2$), L-phenlalanine mustard (L-PAM), and a combination of an alkylating agent and actinomycin-D (Table 2). Single agents were used in most early perfusions. Recommended doses of agents used by us is shown in Table 3, and by other investigators in Table 4. Doxorubicin was used in two cases, but neither patient had a clinical response. This drug is partially precipitated by heparin, which limits its use in regional perfusion.

Table 2. Drugs used in 122 patients with soft tissue sarcoma of limb.

	Number patients	
Drug	First perfusion	Subsequent perfusion
Nitrogen mustard (HN$_2$)	30	4
L-Phenylalanine mustard (L-PAM)	38	1
L-PAM, actinomycin D	20	4
L-PAM, TSPA	3	2
L-PAM, HN$_2$, actinomycin D	18	1
L-PAM, TSPA, actinomycin D	2	1
HN$_2$, actinomycin D	1	—
Doxorubicin	2	—
Misc. and other combinations	8	1
Total	122	14

Table 3. Tulane dosage for hyperthermic perfusion for limb sarcoma.

	Upper limb		Lower limb	
I.A. Line	Range	Max	Range	Max
Single drug	mg/kg	mg	mg/kg	mg
Melphalan	0.6—1.0	65	0.8—1.2	100
HN$_2$	0.3—0.6	30	0.4—0.8	40
Cisplatin	1.0—2.0	100	1.0—4.0	150
Multiple drugs				
Melphalan	0.4—0.7	45	0.5—0.8	60
and TSPA	0.2—0.3	25	0.5—0.9	35
Melphalan	0.5—0.7	45	0.5—0.9	60
Act. D,	0.006—0.01	0.5	0.008—0.012	0.75
and HN$_2$	0.07—0.11	10	0.08—0.15	12

Fractional intra-arterial line doses reservoir volume 500—700 cc, $\frac{1}{2}$ whole blood, $\frac{1}{2}$ balanced electrolyte solution.
Limb temperatures approximately 40°C.

Results of Treatment

The results of treatment of soft tissue sarcoma of the limb in 122 patients from 1957 to 1980 are summarized in Table 5. Of 56 patients with Stage I disease who were treated with perfusion and wide excision, 12 (21%) developed local recurrence. Ten of these patients had lesions larger than 5 cm in diameter, four were controlled by further operations, three with wide excision, and one with amputation. The 5- and 10-year cummulative survival rates for these patients were both 64.9%. Four patients had amputations early in the series, at a time when amputation was standard treatment. As results improved, wide excision was substituted for amputation. Adjuvant therapy after resection was not routinely used; however, five patients had

115

Table 4. Reported dosage for hyperthermic perfusion limb sarcoma.

Investigator	Drug	Limb/Dosage	Route
Fletcher	CDDP	Arm 6.0 mg/kg Leg 6.3 mg/kg	PR 1/2 dose at q. 5 min intervals
De Filippo	CDDP	3, 2 mg/kg	PR divided doses
Dildolkar	DTIC	Arm 1 gm/M2 Leg 2 gm/M2	PR given in 3—4 divided doses q. 5 min
Aigner	L-PAM CDDP	10 mg/L 15 mg/L	IA infusion PR single dose
Wieberdink	L-PAM Doxorubicin Doxorubicin and L-PAM	10 mg/L 10 mg/L 5—20 mg/L 4—13 mg/L	IA infusion
Schraffordt–Koops	L-PAM Dactinomycin	Arm 0.5—0.7 mg/kg Leg 1.0—1.5 mg/kg Arm 0.006 mg/kg Leg 0.014 mg/kg	PR single dose
McBride	L-PAM Dactinomycin	Arm 0.7 mg/kg Leg 1.3 mg/kg Arm 0.02 mg/kg Leg 0.03 mg/kg	PR single dose

PR = pump reservoir; IA = intra-arterial line; L = liter of limb volume; temperature approximately 40°C.

Table 5. Results of treatment by regional perfusion in 122 patients with limb soft tissue sarcoma, 1957—1980.

Stage and therapy	Patients treated	Survival, cumulative (%)		
		5 Years	10 Years	15 Years
Localized	72			
Primary lesion, perfused and resected	56	64.9	64.9	51.6
Primary lesion, perfusion alone	16	0	0	0
Regional	36			
Local recurrent lesion, perfused and resected	11	90	75	66
Local recurrent lesion, perfusion alone	3	33.4	33.4	33.4
Primary lesion with regional metastases, perfused and resected	10	15.6	0	0
Local recurrence and regional metastases, perfused and resected	12	43.9	35.9	35.9
Distant disease Limb perfusion and/or resection for palliation	14	0	—	—

irradiation in the immediate pre- or postperfusion period, one had intra-arterial chemotherapy, and one received adjuvant immunotherapy with *bacillus Calmette-Guerin* (BCG).

The response in the patients who had bone involvement treated with regional perfusion alone was poor. The Ewing's sarcoma responded well, but recurred within 1 year, while patients with osteogenic sarcoma usually had good relief of pain; we had no long-term control of patients with primary bone sarcomas.

Tumor size is one of the best prognostic indicators for soft tissue sarcoma, except for synovial cell sarcoma. Of 50 patients having evaluable tumor sizes with complete excision following perfusion of the primary tumor, there is a significant difference in survival rates for all tumor types when compared by size. For tumors measuring up to 20 cm^2, 85% of the patients are living with no evidence of disease at 3 or more years. For tumors between 20 and 40 cm^2, the 3-year disease-free survival is 58%, and for tumors more than 40 cm^2, it is 50%.

When the tumor is localized, complete wide soft tissue resection is always desirable, but often not possible, as a limb-sparing procedure. In the group of 86 patients with localized tumors, 67 were resected just prior to, at the time of, or in the immediate postperfusion period. Of the 19 never resected, two had complete regression, and three had excellent partial responses, but all, except one patient, eventually had fatal progression of the disease.

The marked difference in survival for local recurrent lesions compared to primary lesions is compatible with sarcoma behavior. Sarcomas that evolve slowly, recur locally, and metastasize late have a higher survival rate in the early years. The 5- and 10-year survival rates for 11 patients with recurrent tumors treated by perfusion and resection were 90 and 75%, respectively. The cumulative survival rate for 22 patients with regional metastases is dependent partly on the natural biologic characteristics of soft tissue sarcoma (Table 5). Twelve patients with indolent lesions coming to diagnosis and with regional metastases following a local recurrence had a better survival rate (44 and 36%, respectively, at 5 and 10 years) compared to 15.6% at 5 years and 0% at 10 years for patients with primary and regional spread of disease at diagnosis.

Approximately 55% of the patients had a wide excision prior to or concurrent with perfusions. In the remaining 51 patients with lesions measurable after perfusion, 18 underwent delayed therapeutic excision, and 33 never had resection (Table 6). The overall objective response rate in patients with delayed or unresected tumor was 62.5%. The three patients who achieved a complete regression were a 55-year-old woman with a large primary hemangiosarcoma of the arm, a 2-year-old girl with rhabdomyosarcoma of the calf, and a 35-year-old man with a multifocal fibrosarcoma of the foot. They remained without evidence of tumor for 45, 23, and 2 months, respectively, before recurrence and metastases led to death at 96, 39, and 23 months, respectively.

Table 6. Following regional chemotherapy perfusion delayed excision or no excision results of treatment of leg perfusion in 51 patients.

	Extent of disease			
	Localized	Regional	Regional and distant	Total
Number of patients treated	28	11	12	51
Response				
None	9	2	6	17
<50%	12	4	5	21
>50%	5	1	0	6
Complete	2	1	0	3
Not evaluated	0	3	1	4
Total	19/28 = 68%	6/8 = 75%	6/11 = 55%	29/47 = 62%

Of the various tissue types treated by perfusion and excision, the best response rate occurred in patients with synovial sarcoma. Of six patients with Stage I disease, five have no evidence of disease and good functioning limbs at more than 10 years post-treatment. One living at 12 years had a recurrence excised at 5 years. One example is a 21-year-old woman who was an active volley ball player, had synovial sarcoma of the knee, and refused amputation. This patient responded well to perfusion with melphalan, with a more than 50% decrease in tumor mass. A wide excision of the lateral knee joint and reconstruction 1 month later provided her with a good knee joint, enabling her to return to normal activity (figure 3). She remains living and well at present, 11 years post-treatment.

One example of good palliation with presentation of a useful limb in a 78-year-old woman with undifferentiated sarcoma developing in the lateral surface of the knee is seen in figure 4. A good response was seen following a melphalan perfusion, permitting a wide local excision 14 days later, with repair with a split thickness skin graft. Local control was achieved, but the patient died 19 months post-treatment from pulmonary metastases.

In the entire series, 39 patients had varying degrees of pain; of 18 with intense or moderate pain, 9 had moderate-to-dramatic relief following perfusion.

Deaths and Complications

While regional chemotherapy by isolated limb perfusion is not without risk, it is generally well tolerated and, most importantly, usually does not produce systemic toxicity precluding further chemotherapy. There were only two treatment-related deaths in 122 patients; one was due to cardiac arrest during surgery, and the second was due to multiple pulmonary emboli and massive pulmonary infarct 5 weeks following perfusion and resection.

Three amputations were performed as a result of complications of therapy, all early in the development of the technique prior to 1962; five patients had therapeutic amputation. Therefore, only 8 (7%) of 122 patients lost their limbs, using regional hyperthermic perfusion for the treatment of limb soft tissue sarcoma.

Observations and Conclusions

The goal of the treatment of extremity soft tissue sarcoma is to obtain local and regional control to the disease, with the preservation of limb function, while preserving overall survival. Chemotherapy by regional hyperthermic perfusion combined with wide excision is an effective limb-sparing procedure. Regional perfusion however should not be viewed as just a means of delivering a higher regional dose of chemotherapy. It is also important to understand that regional perfusion improves the pharmacokinetics and pharmacodynamics of drug delivery, which is potentiated by the effects of hyperthermia and hyperoxygenation. Since 1957 at Tulane University School of Medicine, limb salvage for 122 patients is better than 93%, and the 10-year survival rate is 65%. The multidisciplinary approach, as popularized by Eilber and Morton, using preoperative intra-arterial chemotherapy and rapid fraction radiotherapy followed by wide excision and adjuvant chemotherapy, has lowered the local recurrence rate to 3 to 5%, but at the expense of a relatively high complication rate. Even though a limb-salvage rate of 90% for patients has been achieved, the 3-year survival rate remains only 68%. Local recurrence rates, using regional perfusion, vary between 9 and 20%, and it is encouraging that the local recurrence rate, using cisplatin in one series, has been completely prevented. Further improvement of the perfusion technique may result from combining melphalan and cisplatin, which will provide good activity against most of the individual types of soft tissue sarcoma.

Figure 3. 21-Year-old white woman with synovial sarcoma over left lateral knee of 2-months ▶ duration. A common femoral artery hyperthermic perfusion with 60 mg of melphalan, 0.5 mg of Actinomycin D, and 10 mg of nitrogen mustard was performed on 2/22/79. The mass decreased in size by more than 50%. On 3/21/79 the lateral portion of knee joint including head of fibula was excised. A 1 cm nodule of residual tumor found in lateral joint surface. Patient has had full rehabilitation of her knee and is living and well at present, 11 years postop. treatment. (A) Preperfusion photo of right and left knee. Note swelling on lateral side of left knee. (B) Postperfusion photo prior to excision reducing size of left knee mass. (C) Specimen of left knee resection. Note residual sarcoma in inner surface of lateral knee joint. (D) Anatomical sketch of left knee, flexed, anterior posterior view, patella absent showing approximate original and postperfusion tumor margins and surgical excision margin in broken line.

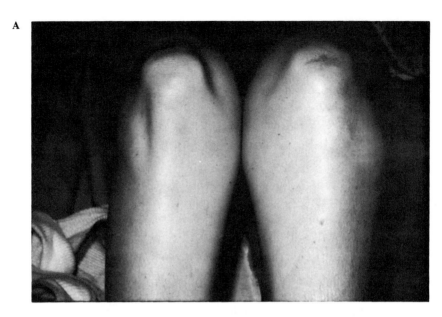

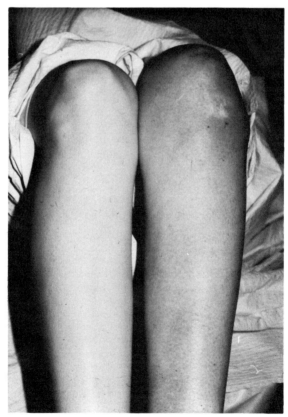

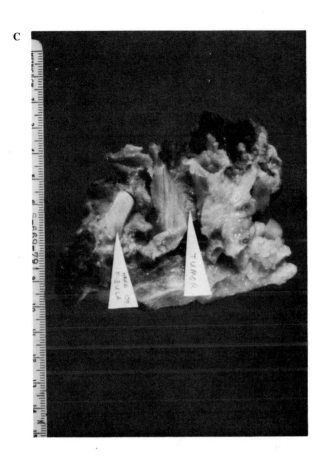

C

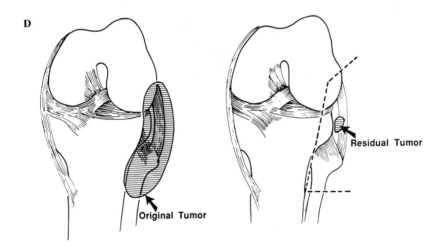

D

Original Tumor

Residual Tumor

121

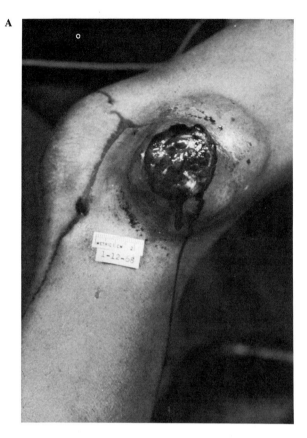

Figure 4. (A) Undifferentiated sarcoma developing on the lateral surface of left knee of a 78-year-old woman. (B) Perfusion with melphalan resulted in regression of tumor, seen 14 days later. (C) Sarcoma was resected, and the defect repaired with a split thickness skin graft. Local control achieved; patient developed pulmonary metastases one year later and died 19 months after initial treatment.

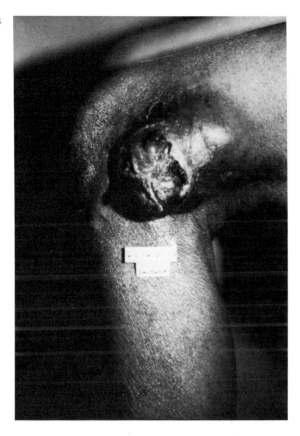

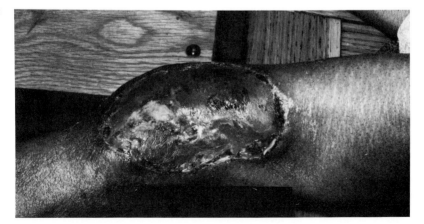

123

Acknowledgments

The authors wish to acknowledge the support in part of the Melville John Jacobson Cancer Research Fund, the Carl Otto Cancer Research Fund, and the Armande Billion Clinical Cancer Research Fund. They wish to recognize the secretarial and editorial assistance of Jessie Brupbacher, Andrew Bird, and Heide Dyer.

References

1. McClay EF: Epidemiology of bone and soft tissue sarcomas. Semin Oncol 16 (4):254—272.
2. Silverberg E, Lubera JA: Cancer statistics. Cancer 38:14—15, 1988.
3. Cadman J, Soule FH, Kelly PJ: Synovial sarcomas: An analysis of 134 tumors. Cancer 18:613—627, 1965.
4. Shieber W, Graham P: An experience with sarcoma of the soft tissues in adults. Surgery 52:295—298, 1962.
5. Castro EB, Hajdu SI, Fortner JG: Surgical therapy of fibrosarcoma of extremities. Arch Surg 107:284—291, 1973.
6. Shiu MH, Castro EB, Hajdu SI, Fortner JG: Surgical treatment of 297 soft tissue sarcomas of the lower extremity. Ann Surg 182:597—602, 1975.
7. Cautin J, McNeer GP, Chu FC, Booker RJ: The problem of local recurrence after treatment of soft tissue sarcoma. Ann Surg 168:47—53, 1968.
8. Simon MA, Spanier SS, Euneking WF: Management of adult soft tissue sarcomas of the extremities. Ann Surg 11:363—402, 1979.
9. Klopp CT, Alford TC, Bateman J, et al.: Fractionated intra-arterial cancer chemotherapy with bis-amine hydrochloride; a preliminary report. Ann Surg 132:811—832, 1950.
10. Bierman HR, Byron RL, Jr, Kelly KH: Therapy of inoperable visceral and regional metastasis by intra-arterial catheterization in man. Cancer Res 11:236, 1951.
11. Creech OJ, Krementz ET, Ryan RT, Winblad JN: Chemotherapy of cancer: Regional perfusion utilizing an extracorporeal circuit. Ann Surg 148:616—632, 1958.
12. Krementz ET: Regional perfusion: Current sophistication, what next? Cancer 57 (3):416—430, 1986.
13. Krementz ET, Carter RD, Sutherland CM, Hutton IM: Chemotherapy of sarcomas of the limbs by regional perfusion. Ann Surg 185 (5), 1977.
14. Krementz ET, Muchmore JH: Soft tissue sarcomas: Behavior and management. Adv Surg 16:147—196, 1983.
15. Carter RD, Faddis DM, Krementz ET, Salwen WA, Puyau FA, Muchmore JH: Treatment of locally advanced breast cancer with regional intra-arterial chemotherapy. Reg Cancer Treat 1:108—111, 1988.
16. Kaulheim G, Gundersen S, Hager B, et al.: Intra-arterial infusion of mitomycin-C in treatment of breast cancer: Occurrence of skin necrosis in irradiated patients. Radiother Oncol 4:127—132, 1985.
17. Auersperg M, Furlan L, Marolt F, et al.: Intra-arterial chemotherapy and radiotherapy in locally advanced cancer of the oral cavity and oropharynx. Int J Radiat Oncol Biol Phys 4:273—277, 1978.
18. Huberman MG: Comparison of systemic chemotherapy with hepatic arterial infusion in metastatic colorectal carcinoma. Semin Oncol 10:238—248, 1983.
19. Oberfield RA: Intra-arterial hepatic infusion chemotherapy in metastatic liver cancer. Semin Oncol 10:206—214, 1983.
20. Kemeny N, Daly J, Reichman B, et al.: Intrahepatic or systemic infusion of fluorodeoxyuri-

dine in patients with liver metastases from colorectal carcinoma. Ann Intern Med 107:459—465, 1987.

21. Eapen L, Stewart D, Danjoux C, et al.: Intra-arterial cisplatin and concurrent radiation for locally advanced bladder cancer. J Clin Oncol 7:230—235, 1989.

22. Shipley WU, Prout GR, Einstein AB, et al.: Treatment of invasive bladder cancer by cisplatin and radiation in patients unsuited for surgery. JAMA 258:931—935, 1987.

23. Eilber FR, Guiliano AE, Huth J, Mirra J, Morton DL: Limb salvage for high-grade soft tissue sarcomas of the extremity: Experience at the University of California, Los Angeles. Cancer Treat Symp 3:49—57, 1985.

24. Mantravadi RV, Trippon MJ, Patel MS, Walker MJ, Das Gupta TK: Limb salvage in extremity soft-tissue sarcoma: Combined modality therapy. Radiology 152:523—526, 1984.

25. Denton JW, Dunham WK, Salter M, Urist NM, Balch CM: Pre-operative regional chemotherapy and rapid-fraction irradiation for sarcomas of the soft tissue and bone. Surg Gynecol Obstet 158:545—551, 1984.

26. Goodnight JE, Bargar WL, Voegeli T, Blaisdell FW: Limb-sparing surgery for extremity sarcomas after pre-operative intra-arterial doxorubicin and radiation therapy. Am J Surg 150:109—113, 1985.

27. Stephens FO, Tattersall MHN, Marsden W, Waugh RC, Green D, McCarthy SW: Regional chemotherapy with the use of cisplatin and doxorubicin as primary treatment for advanced sarcomas in shoulder, pelvis, and thigh. Cancer 60:724—735, 1987.

28. Hoekstra HJ, Heimen SK, Molenaar WM, Oldhoff J: Results of isolated perfusion of malignant soft tissue tumors of the extremities. Cancer 60:1703—1707, 1987.

29. Azzarelli A, Gennari L, Quaglivlo V: Intra-arterial chemotherapy for soft tissue sarcoma of the extremities in management of soft tissue and bone sarcomas. In: Management of soft tissue tumors and bone sarcoma. Van Unnik JA, Van Oosterom AT (eds). New York: Raven Press, 1986.

30. Collins JM: Pharmacologic rationale for regional drug deliver. J Clin Oncol 2:498—504, 1984.

31. Ensminger WD, Gyves JW: Clinical pharmacology of hepatic arterial chemotherapy. Semin Oncol 10:176—182, 1983.

32. Steward DJ, Benjamin RS, Zimmerman S, et al.: Clinical pharmacology of intra-arterial cis-diamminedichloroplatinum (II). Cancer Res 43:917—920, 1983.

33. Garnick MB, Ensminger WD, Israel M: A clinical-pharmacological evaluation of hepatic arterial infusion of adriamycin. Cancer Res 39:4105—4110, 1979.

34. Gyves JW, Stetson P, Ensminger WD, et al.: Hepatic arterial streptozotocin: A clinical pharmacologic study in patients with liver tumors. Cancer Drug Deliv 1:63—66, 1983.

35. Stewart DJ, Mikhael NZ, Nair RC, et al.: Platinum concentrations in human autopsy tumor samples. Am J Clin Oncol (CCT) 11:152—158, 1988.

36. Levin VA, Kabra PM, Freeman–Dove MA: Pharmacokinetics of intracarotid artery ^{14}C-BCNU in the squirrel monkey. J Neurosurg 48:587—593, 1978.

37. Didolkar MS, Kanter PM, Baffi RR, et al.: Comparison of regional versus systemic chemotherapy with adriamycin. Ann Surg 187:332—336, 1978.

38. Anderson LL, Collings GJ, Ojima Y, et al.: A study of the distribution of methotrexate in human tissues and tumors. Cancer Res 30:1344—1348, 1970.

39. Erjavea M, Auersperg M, Jez T: Quantitation of ^{99m}TC bleomycin uptake in head and neck tumors. IRCS (J) Med Sci 2:1560, 1974.

40. Savaraj N, Lu K, Feun LG, et al.: Comparison of CNS penetration, tissue distribution, and pharmacology of VP16-213 by intracarotid and intravenous administration in dogs. Cancer Invest 5:11—16, 1987.

41. Wallace S, Chuang VP, Carrasco H, et al.: Physioanatomic concepts and radiologic techniques for intra-arterial delivery of therapeutic agents. Cancer Bull 36:6—14, 1984.

42. Muchmore JH, Carter RD, Krementz ET: Regional perfusion for malignant melanoma and soft tissue sarcoma: A review. Cancer Invest 3 (2):129—143, 1985.

125

43. Cavaliere R, Calabro A, DiFillippo F, Carlini S, Giannavelli D: Prognostic parameters in limb recurrent melanoma treated with hyperthermic antiblastic perfusion. Conference on Advances in Regional Cancer Therapy, Ulm, Federal Republic of German, G7 (Abstr): 163, 1987.
44. Stehlin JS, Greeff PJ, deIpolyi PD, Giovanella BC, Klein G, McGaff CJ, Jr, Davis B, Williams LJ, Natelson EA, Anderson RF: Heat as an adjuvant in the treatment of advanced melanoma. An immune stimulant? Houston Med J 4:61, 1988.
45. Flaherty JH, Weisfeldt ML: Reperfusion injury. Free Radic Biol Med 5:409—419, 1988.
46. Krementz ET, Ryan RF, Muchmore JH, Carter RD, Sutherland CM, Reed RJ: Hyper-thermic regional perfusion for melanoma of the limbs. In: Cutaneous melanoma, clinical management and treatment. Balch CM, Milton G (eds). Philadelphia: JB Lippincott, in press.

10. Thermochemotherapy for Soft Tissue Sarcomas

F. Di Filippo, C. Botti, D. Giannarelli, F. Graziano, S. Carlini,
F. Cavaliere, and R. Cavaliere

Introduction

Many years ago, several in vitro and in vivo experimental studies demonstrated the selective heat sensitivity of cancer cells. The first clinical applications of hyperthermia then confirmed its effectiveness for treating cancer [1-5].

Since then, many techniques have been developed to carry out loco-regional and systemic hyperthermia in clinical oncology. More recently, nonionizing energies (microwaves, radiofrequencies, and ultrasounds) have also been used for loco-regional therapy [6,7].

In spite of recent technological advances in heat transfer and the standardization of hyperthermic treatments, two major limitations hamper the therapeutic effectiveness of hyperthermia: (a) difficulty in achieving a homogeneous cytotoxic temperature while simultaneously sparing the normal tissue; and (b) thermal resistance [8,9].

As demonstrated in experimental and clinical studies, these limitations have been partially overcome by combining hyperthermia with either radio- or chemotherapy, combinations which have a synergistic effect in killing tumor cells [10-14].

Thermochemotherapy has been employed for the loco-regional and systemic treatment of a large variety of solid human tumors.

This chapter focuses on the role of thermochemotherapy for treating soft tissue sarcomas.

Interactions of Hyperthermia and Chemotherapy

Hyperthermia has a tumor cell-specific cytotoxic effect by means of two mechanisms. The first is a direct action of the heat on some cellular components or functions (membrane, cytoskeleton, lysosomes, respiration, DNA, RNA, protein synthesis, etc.), producing often irreversible damage [15]. The second is mediated by heat-induced modifications of the tumor

Pinedo, H.M., Verweij, J., and H.D. Suit (eds.): Soft Tissue Sarcomas: New Developments in
the Multidisciplinary Approach to Treatment. © *1991 Kluwer Academic Publishers, Boston.*
ISBN: 0-7923-1139-6. All rights reserved.

Table 1. Tumor blood flow modifiers.

Drugs changing vessel wall tension
— Vasoactive agents
— Norepinephrine
— Angiotensin-II
— 5-Hydroxytriptamine
— Hydralazine
Drugs changing blood viscosity
— Glucose
— Calcium entry blocking agents

microcirculation [16-18], which, in turn, worsens hypoxia and lowers the pH, enhancing the direct cytotoxic effect of hyperthermia.

Some antineoplastic drugs enhance the efficacy of heat in cancer killing by increasing the number of intracellular heat shock proteins, correlating with the appearance and decay of thermotolerance [19,20]. Five-thio-D-glucose and lonidamine, inhibitors of glucose metabolism, increase hyperthermia-induced cytotoxicity [21,22]; also, the quercitin-inhibiting lactate transport improves the tumoricidal effect of heat, most likely by exacerbating tumor cell acidosis [23-26].

Tumor blood flow heterogeneity is detrimental for the hyperthermic treatment of tumors, since it does not permit uniform tumor heating. The hyperthermic effect would be significantly greater if agents that selectively modify the tumor blood flow were employed, making the treatment more uniform.

Some of the drugs that appear able to selectively modify tumor circulation, acting directly on the vessels and indirectly on the blood viscosity and therefore improving the homogeneity of the heating, are listed in Table 1 [27].

The therapeutic efficacy of hyperthermia is biologically limited by thermoresistance expressed by some cell clones, which may be overcome with different therapeutic combinations. Numerous in vitro and in vivo studies have shown that the hyperthermia-chemotherapy combination may result in an additive or synergistic effect, increasing the tumor response obtained by the single methods [28].

Not all the mechanisms of the hyperthermia-chemotherapy interactions are known, but the many experimental studies conducted thus far have permitted identification of some of the pharmacokinetic and pharmacodynamic modifications that explain the greater efficacy of the hyperthermia-chemotherapy combination (Table 2).

Many enzymatic reactions are temperature dependent because of either an increased metabolic activation or inactivation. For example, for mitomycin-C a greater production of active alkylating metabolites can be observed at high temperatures, exactly opposite to what occurs with cyclophosphamide [29,30].

128

Table 2. Interactions of hyperthermia and chemotherapy.

Enzymatic changes
Tumor drug uptake
— blood flow
— membrane permeability
Protein binding
DNA Effects
— increased alkylation
— increased oxygen radical production
— reduced sublethal damage repair

It has been shown experimentally that hyperthermia increases tumor cell drug uptake by means of tumor blood flow and cellular membrane changes. The initial increase in temperature induces greater tumor blood flow, which augments the quantity of drug reaching the tumor. After further increase of temperature, the microcirculation collapses, and the drug is "trapped" in the tumor. The intracellular drug uptake may be even more facilitated by the increased permeability of the tumor cell membrane. In fact, hyperthermia can increase the intracellular concentration of cisplatin in cisplatin-sensitive and in resistant CHO cell strains [31] and cause a greater drug accumulation in P388 leukemia cells than in murine bone marrow cells [32].

Hyperthermia also inhibits some antineoplastic drugs in the formation of drug-protein complexes. This phenomenon is extremely important for the cytotoxic effects of the drug because only the nonprotein-bound and therefore diffusible fraction can react with target cells. Once the drug has penetrated into the tumor cell, the combined hyperthermia-drug effect can greatly damage the DNA, with subsequent cell death. Single-strand DNA breakage has been reported for many antineoplastic drugs [33-36]. In studies conducted by Johnson and Pavelec, damage to the DNA by thiotepa occurred with a modest energy activation, indicating that chemotherapy can complement the hyperthermic activity, making a moderate thermal dose necessary in order to obtain an isoeffect [37].

Two other mechanisms can explain the synergistic effect of the hyperthermia-chemotherapy combination. The first is a direct inhibition of hyperthermia on the polymerase beta enzyme responsible for sublethal DNA damage repair from chemotherapy [38]. The second is that both hyperthermia and some cytotoxic drugs possess an alkylating effect on DNA. The formation of oxygen radicals can be increased by the depletion of cellular gluthathione, which functions as an oxygen radical scavanger [39,40].

These interactions of hyperthermia and chemotherapy have not been observed for all antineoplastic drugs, many of which behave nonhomogeneously with heat.

Hahn classified the drugs into four categories according to their interactions with heat [35,41-46].

129

Classes	Agents
1. Drugs showing no threshold effect	thiotepa, nitrosoureas, mitomycin-C, cisplatin
2. Drugs showing marked threshold effects	doxorubicin, bleomycin, actinomycin D
3. Thermosensitizers	cysteamine, amphotericin B, AET, lidocaine, polyamine
4. Drugs showing no interaction with heat	antimetabolites, vincristine, vinblastine

Cytotoxic agents that show a greater linear cytotoxicity with increasing temperatures belong to the first category [24,25,37,41,42,47,48]. The second includes drugs that do not exhibit linear cytotoxicity with heat, but show a threshold temperature effect at 42 to 43°C [10-17, 46]. The third group of heat-interactive drugs presents no cytotoxicity at 37°C, but becomes tumoricidal at higher temperatures [43,45]. The fourth group shows no changes in cytotoxicity at a 37 to 45°C range [25,43,46].

Biological response modifiers (BRMs) demonstrating an antineoplastic activity and showing promising results have recently been employed in clinical practice. Some of these have been used in experimental studies in association with hyperthermia: interferon [49], the tumor necrosis factor (TNF) [50-52], and interleukin-2 (IL-2) with or without TNF [53]. In all of the experiments, the combination of hyperthermia with BRMs has provided better responses than those obtained with single methods.

The interactions between hyperthermia and chemotherapy are quite complex and can only result in a synergistic effect if the modalities are combined appropriately. Many in vitro and in vivo experiments have demonstrated that the most important factors concerning synergism are the temperature level, treatment sequence, and timing. Some drugs, such as cisplatin and L-phenyl alanine mustard (L-PAM, melphalan), only show a synergistic effect at 42°C [54] and only with the simultaneous application of heat. Other timing sequences produce only an additive or adverse effect [47,54].

These experimental results have been confirmed clinically with hyperthermic antiblastic perfusion (H.A.P.): the best results being achieved at a temperature of 41.5°C or more and with a standard or higher than standard drug dosage [55].

Preclinical Studies

The majority of data on the interactions between hyperthermia and chemotherapy have been obtained in in vitro studies employing various tumor cell lines. These studies present two distinct limits: (1) differences in the conditions between in vitro and in vivo studies in animals, with totally diverse pharmacokinetic and pharmacodynamic conditions (tumor vascularization,

Table 3. Thermochemotherapy for soft tissue sarcoma: preclinical studies.

Author	Drug	Schedule (°C)	Schedule (min)	Effect uptake	Effect cytotoxic
Marijnissen (1988)	Photophrin	44	30	=	↑
Kallinowsky (1989)	TNF	42—44	40		↑
Pfeffer (1989)	Cisplatin	43	30	↑	↑
Nishiue (1989)	Cisplatin	43	30		↑
George (1989)	Trimeprazine + Melphalan	42	60	=	↑
Baba (1989)	Doxorubicin	41.5	120	=	↑

metabolic modifications, total body drug clearance, etc.), and (2) the possible diverse sensitivity of different tumors with regard to the combined treatment.

We therefore wanted to established whether similar interactions between hyperthermia and chemotherapy were observed in vivo in an animal model, using a sarcoma.

In the six experimental studies reported in Table 3, the association of hyperthermia and chemotherapy always was more effective than the use of both modalities separately.

Interesting results have been obtained with new drugs, such as photophrin and TNF, both able to damage the tumor microcirculation, thereby enhancing the hyperthermic effect. Tumor control rates of 40 to 50% have been reported [50,56].

With regard to the combination with conventional antiblastic drugs (cisplatin, L-PAM), some of the factors involved in synergism have been confirmed in vivo: the combination of hyperthermia and chemotherapy is more effective due to the enhanced tumor drug uptake at high temperatures with an increase of DNA cross-linking by cisplatin [57]. It has also been confirmed that only the simultaneous administration of hyperthermia and chemotherapy can offer any advantage [58].

Applying a drug able to increase the membrane permeability (Trimeprazine), George et al. [59] obtained a 60% cure rate in animals treated with hyperthermia and L-PAM, thus confirming the important role of the altered permeability of the tumor cell membrane. This is quite important when we consider that L-PAM has never been effective for treating sarcomas.

Baba observed a thermal enhancement ratio (TER) of 1.8 in tumor growth delay, applying doxorubicin (DX), 5 mg/kg at 41.5°C. However, the systemic administration of high DX doses caused a TER increase (1.4 to 1.8) in terms of LD_{50} as well, thus diminishing the therapeutic gain [60].

Techniques

Several techniques have been developed for local, regional, and whole body hyperthermic treatments. Loco-regional heating has been clinically carried out with hyperthermic perfusion, ultrasounds, and electromagnetic waves.

The technique of hyperthermic perfusion has been previously described. In brief, the blood circulates in an extracorporeal circuit equipped with an oxygenator, a pump, and a heat exchanger: the blood acting as a heat transfer in the tumor region.

New devices have recently been developed that are able to produce hyperthermia with different sources: (a) ultrasounds operating at a frequency range of 0.3 to 6 MHz; and (b) electromagnetic waves (microwaves or radio frequencies) at a 13 to 2,450 MHz range.

Devices applying alternating electromagnetic fields can produce heat either by induction of electrical currents (inductive system) or by direct coupling of electromagnetic currents between the applicators encompassing the tissue to be heated (capacitive system). Clinical applications have demonstrated that many of these devices are quite effective for heating superficial lesions, but none developed for deep heating are yet completely reliable.

Whole body hyperthermia techniques have been extensively reported by Milligan [61]. At present, three different techniques for delivering systemic hyperthermia are used. The first utilizes direct contact between the skin and some heat-transporting vehicles, such as water, wax, or air. The second employs body surface irradiation with nonionizing energies. The third technique is extracorporeal perfusion, which appears to be the most effective because it permits reaching a 41.5 to 41.8°C temperature within 30 to 39 minutes.

Local Hyperthermia by Perfusion

Experience at the Regina Elena National Cancer Institute

Our first experiences with H.A.P. as a single treatment modality for soft tissue limb sarcomas were previously described in the 1989 issue of *Treatment of Soft Tissue Sarcomas*.

A total of 80 patients were treated with this technique between 1971 and December 1989. Eight patients presented with visceral metastases as well as with local relapses and were therefore not included in any of the treat-

Variables	Treatment protocol (No. of patients)		
	HAP + surgery	HAP + i.a. DX infusion + surgery	HAP + RT + surgery
Age			
≤50 years	12	9	12
> 50 years	21	8	8
Sex			
Male	20	11	10
Female	13	6	10
No. of previous recurrences			
0	15	7	10
1	7	5	5
≥2	11	5	5
Site			
Proximal	19	9	9
Distal	14	8	11
Grade			
I—II	23	8	12
III	10	9	8
Tumor stage			
T1	3	3	3
T2	14	8	12
T3	16	6	5
Node stage			
N0	29	16	19
N1	4	1	1
Disease stage			
I	3	3	2
II	4	2	8
III	10	7	5
IVA	16	5	5

ment protocols. Two treatment-related deaths occurred: one caused by a massive hemorrhage after iliac artery rupture, and the other by myocardial infarction.

Table 4 presents the patient characteristics according to the treatment protocol adopted. At the time of the referral, 48 out of 70 patients (68.5%) had Stage III-IVA disease, and 38 (54.2%) had recurrences of previously treated sarcomas. Most of the patients had developed multiple recurrences (as many as five in several cases) after either surgery alone or multimodality treatments.

The technique of limb perfusion has been previously described [63]. The drug is administered when the limb reaches a temperature of 41.5°C. To avoid major complications, the muscle temperature never exceeds 41.8°C.

Melphalan (0.8 mg/kg of body weight [b.w.]) and actinomycin D (DACT or dactinomycin; 0.015 mg/kg b.w.) were the drugs used in the first series of 50 patients. Twenty-two other patients were treated with different dosages and schedules of cisplatin (2.5, 3.2, and 5.0 mg/kg b.w.). In the remaining eight patients, different schedules and dosages of DX (1.0, 1.2, 1.4, and 1.6 mg/kg b.w.) were used.

All of the 70 patients were treated with additional therapy according to different protocols as follows: (1) H.A.P. plus surgery, (2) H.A.P. plus intra-arterial (i.a.) DX plus surgery, or (3) H.A.P. plus radiotherapy plus surgery.

The i.a. DX infusion was generally initiated within 10 days after the H.A.P. (3 cycles, 10 mg/kg for 10 days each, administered at 10-day intervals, followed by delayed surgery). Radiotherapy was given by an external beam source within 4 weeks after the H.A.P. All the patients received a dosage that varied between 45 and 65 Gy, depending on local tolerance. Delayed surgery was performed 3 to 4 weeks later.

Regarding morbidity, only two amputations were directly related to the perfusion in the group treated with H.A.P. plus surgery: one patient treated with H.A.P. plus i.a. DX infusion plus surgery developed arteritis with progressive arterial insufficiency, requiring amputation 14 months after the perfusion; and another, treated with H.A.P. plus radiotherapy and surgery, developed a postactinic necrosis of the femur, requiring amputation 30 months after the perfusion. Four patients had venous thrombosis, which promptly recovered after standard therapy. Chronic renal insufficiency and moderate, but irreversible, neuropathy occurred in two patients treated with high-dose cisplatin (5.0 mg/kg b.w.) during the H.A.P. Since both local and systemic toxicity appeared to be strictly dose related, 3.2 mg/kg b.w. appears to be a safe dose for temperatures that do not exceed 41.5°C [63].

The patient's sex, age, tumor site, T and N staging (according to the AJC classification), the type of therapeutic protocol, and the histological tumor grade were recorded in a computerized data base. The median follow-up was 39 months (range, 3 to 183 months). Survival was calculated from the time of the H.A.P.

The patients were evaluated in terms of local control, percentage of conservative treatments carried out, and local disease-free, distant disease-free, and overall survival rates. For the statistical analysis, the Kaplan Meier method was used. Finally, a multivariate analysis was made using the treatment protocol as the prognostic factor to test for it in association with the overall survival, as the end point.

Table 5 shows the results of the treatment in terms of 5-year loco-regional control. Treatments with H.A.P. plus surgery and H.A.P. plus DX infusion plus surgery provided unsatisfactory results, while better loco-regional control was achieved when radiotherapy was administered between perfusion and surgery. The greater effectiveness of this protocol also permitted performing a higher rate of conservative surgery (Table 6). In addition, limb functionality was not impaired by these multistep treatments.

When all the patients were evaluated, regardless of the treatment, the disease-free, the distant disease-free, and the overall 5-year survival rates were 44.1, 57.1, and 59.6%, respectively.

Table 5. Five-year loco-regional control according to treatment protocol.

Treatment Protocol	%
H.A.P. plus surgery	63.1
H.A.P. plus i.a. DX infusion plus surgery	65.7
H.A.P. plus RT plus surgery	93.3

Table 6. Percentage of conservative surgery according to treatment protocol.

Protocol	Conservative surgery		Demolitive surgery	
H.A.P. plus surgery	19/33	(57.6%)	14/33	(42.4%)
H.A.P. plus i.a. DX infusion plus surgery	15/16	(93.7%)	1/16*	(6.3%)
H.A.P. plus RT plus surgery	19/19**	(100%)	—	

* One patient excluded because of amputation for progressive arteritis, 14 months after H.A.P.
** One patient excluded because of amputation for postactinic necrosis, 30 months after H.A.P.

As Table 7 shows, there tends to be a poorer overall survival, a shorter disease-free interval, and less time to distant recurrences in patients affected with T_3 or multiple recurrent tumors and in those submitted to the H.A.P. plus surgery protocol.

The Cox proportional hazard model was used to analyze the survival times (Table 8). This analysis shows the importance of the tumor size, the number of recurrences before the perfusion, and the protocol adopted, as independent predictors of survival.

Other Clinical Investigations

The results of eight studies employing H.A.P. for the treatment of soft tissue sarcoma are summarized in Table 9. It is readily apparent that the patient characteristics and the protocols employed are different. However, the results should be interpreted in the light of the following: (1) different classification systems have been used, as the patients were not always stratified according to the disease stage and status (primary or recurrent) before the perfusion; (2) the overall, disease-free and distant disease-free survival rates are not always reported; (3) the temperatures applied during the perfusion are not homogeneous and vary between 38 and 41°C; and (4) the treatment schedules have been conducted in different steps: in some cases H.A.P. was performed after the surgical removal of the primary tumor, while in other cases the treatment was carried out in a neoadjuvant setting.

Lethi et al. [64] and Stehlin et al. [65], after H.A.P. administration, used radiotherapy (30 and 50 Gy, respectively) prior to surgery. In addition, the

135

Table 7. Univariate analysis of prognostic variables.

Variable	No. of patients	Actuarial 5 yr. 05%	P value	Actuarial 5 yr. DFS%	P value	Actuarial 5 yr. DDFS%	P value
Age							
≤50 yrs	33	50.6	0.36	45.4	0.76	49.4	0.43
>50 yrs	37	66.9		44.9		63.2	
Sex							
Male	41	57.6	0.87	51.3	0.39	60.9	0.58
Female	29	60.8		40.5		54.1	
Site							
Proximal	37	57.4	0.89	43.3	0.63	58.6	0.69
Distal	33	66.8		47.8		54.3	
Grade							
I—II	43	54.1	0.47	49.2	0.62	56.9	0.80
III	27	67.2		39.2		57.3	

	n						
Tumor stage							
T1	9	75		50		75	
T2	34	75.4		58.4		70.1	
T3	27	36.8	0.02	30	0.08	36.4	0.02
Node stage							
N0	64	59.5		43.7		56.7	
N1	6	60	0.70	33.3	0.43	60	0.89
No. of previous relapses							
0	32	67.5		48.8		63.5	
1	17	55.6		52.2		60	
≥2	21	47.3	0.06	30.2	0.12	42.4	0.15
Treatment protocol							
HAP + surgery	33	48		35.6		44.3	
HAP + i.a. DX							
Infusion + surgery	17	73.3		46.7		66.7	
HAP + RT + surgery	20	70	0.10	68.1	0.08	75.4	0.04
Surgery							
Amputation	17	48.8		45.4		45.4	
Limb sparing	53	63.9	0.07	45.4	0.36	61.6	0.07

OS = overall survival; DFS = disease-free survival; DDFS = distant disease-free survival.

Table 8. Multivariate analysis (Cox model) of prognostic variables (overall survival).

Variables	Initial p-value	Final p-value	Goodness of fit
Age	0.36	. .	
Sex	0.87	. .	
Site	0.89	. .	
Grade	0.47	. .	$p = 0.01$
T	0.02	0.02	
N	0.70		
No. of previous relapses	0.06	0.09	
Treatment protocol	0.10	0.06	
Surgery	0.09	. .	

tumor was not always excised after the H.A.P., although all the authors agree that surgery should be performed after the perfusion, as it permits conservative rather than ablative surgery.

In spite of the above mentioned difficulties, some positive conclusions can be made from comparing the different results obtained with H.A.P. This technique, used either alone or in combination with radiotherapy, has permitted a high rate of conservative surgery (94 to 100%). The low incidence of recurrences (7 to 21%), even in cases where demolitive surgery was not performed, points to the effectiveness of H.A.P. for loco-regional disease control. Finally, a 69 to 75% 5-year survival rate is quite satisfactory when considering the high-risk population treated.

Local Hypertyhermia by Nonionizing Energies

For treating superficial and deep lesions, local hyperthermia by nonionizing energies has been extensively used, primarily in association with radiotherapy. However, only a few reports have been published on the thermochemotherapeutic treatment of soft tissue sarcomas (Table 10).

Jabboury et al. treated 12 advanced soft tissue sarcoma patients for a total of 20 lesions, half of which recurred after definitive radiotherapy [66]. Thirteen lesions were superficial, and seven were deep seated. Hyperthermia was carried out with radio frequencies and/or ultrasounds. Seven lesions were treated with hyperthermia alone, whereas chemotherapy (cisplatin) was added to the treatment of 13 lesions. A temperature of 41.5 to 50°C was reached during the treatments in all the lesions.

An objective response was observed in 50% of the lesions (four complete responses and six partial responses), with a median duration of 4.5 months. Interestingly, objective responses were found in lesions treated at a higher temperature (46.6°C), while lower average temperatures (43.5°C) had been given to the lesions that remained stable.

Issels et al. treated 17 deep-seated soft tissue sarcomas (mean tumor

138

Table 9. Soft tissue sarcoma of the extremities treated with H.A.P. (L-PAM plus DACT).

Authors	Stage	No. of patients	Protocol T (°C)	XRT	Conserv. surgery (%)	Local relapse (%)	Systemic relapse (%)	5-Year survival (%)	Median follow-up (mos)
McBride (1978)	T < 5 cm T > 5 cm	110	39	—	100	15	18	~80 ~80	>60
Stehlin (1984)		65	38.8—40	+(65)	94	—	23	~72.7	?
Lehti (1986)	AJC I—II III—IV	32 32	>40	+(29)	100	11	NE	67	>60
Krementz (1986)	?	56	<41	—	100	21	NE	65	>60
Hoekstra (1987)	I—II III	8 6	38—40	—	94	7	35	69	>156
Kruge (1987)	AJC I—II III—IV	16	?	+(36)	?	11	?	64	?
Lejeune (1988)	T1—T3	14	38—41	+	77	31	38	71 (3 years)	?
Lebredo (1989)	?	46	40	+	98	2	28	?	?

139

Table 10. Loco-regional thermochemotherapy for soft tissue sarcoma: clinical studies.

Author	Drug	No. of patients	Schedule		Effect		
			C°	min.	CR	PR	%OR
Jabboury	Cisplatin	12	41.5—50	60	4	6	50
Issels	Ifosfamide Etoposide	17	40—42.5	30—60	5	4	64
Cavaliere	Cisplatin or Doxorubicin	8	42—43	60	3	1	50

volume 435 cc) [67]. Fourteen were located in the pelvis, one in the abdomen, and two in the proximal thigh. Ten presented with progressive primary disease, and seven recurred after conventional treatment. Chemotherapy (ifosfamide, 1,500 mg/m^2 on days 1 to 5 and etoposide, 100 mg/m^2 on days 1, 3, and 5) was administered together with hyperthermia, the latter given only on days 1 and 5, every 3 to 4 weeks. Treatment was carried out with a device operating at 60 MHz.

Three patients died of progressive disease within 8 months. Complete responses were obtained in five out of 14 patients, and partial responses in four, while four patients remained stable. The median follow-up was 11.2 months.

An analysis of the tumor response showed a good correlation with the thermal parameters: the minimum and maximum tumor temperatures and the thermal dose.

To date, eight soft tissue sarcoma patients have been treated at the Regina Elena National Cancer Institute [68]. Six presented with progressive disease (three after radiotherapy and three after chemotherapy), while two recurred after surgery. The chemotherapeutic regimen (cisplatin, 50 mg/m^2 per week for 4 weeks; and DX, 20 mg/m^2 per week for 6 weeks) was chosen on the basis of the previous chemotherapeutic regimen. Hyperthermia was performed with a device operating at 434 MHz (Sapic S.V. 03 Aeritalia or Enea-Sma), depending on the applicator that better coupled with the lesion to be treated with a 43°C target temperature for 60 minutes.

Three patients obtained a complete response, one had a partial response, and four patients remained stable (median follow-up 5.5 months). Also, in our experience, the response correlated with the minimum and maximum temperature achieved and the thermal dose.

Storm et al., in a multicentric trial of magnetic induction hyperthermia (radio frequencies), treated 130 soft tissue sarcoma patients with heat combined with chemo- or radiotherapy [69]. Objective responses were obtained in 23% of the patients, although the treatments (thermoradio- or thermochemotherapy) responsible for the responses are not specified. It is interesting that when combined with hyperthermia, the same chemo-

Table 11. Systemic thermochemotherapy for soft tissue sarcoma.

Author	No. of patients	Technique	Protocol		Response			Duration (mos)
			HT	CT	CR	PR	S	
Parks et al. (1980)	1	EC41.5-42×5h	Cx	CDDP	—	—	—	—
Herman et al. (1982)	3	EC-WB42-42.5× 2.5-3h	Cx	CDDP or BCNU	—	1	—	2
Barlogie et al. (1979)	1	WB41.9-42×4h	Cx	VP-16	—	1	—	—
Pettigrew et al. (1977)	2	WAX40-41×2h	Cx	—	—	—	—	—
Bull et al. (1986)	16	EC-WB41.8×2h	Cx	BCNU	1	4	—	4
Gerard et al. (1984)	11	WB41.8-43×2h	Cx	DX CTX	2	2	—	12.3
Robins (1989)	2	HRD40.5(75)	Cx	IFN	—	—	2	19—39

therapy treatment caused a tumor regression in previously nonresponding patients.

Systemic Thermochemotherapy

Systemic thermochemotherapy has infrequently also been used in the treatment of metastatic soft tissue sarcomas. Whole body hyperthermia has been carried out by either extracorporeal circulation, with blankets in which hot water circulates, or with heat radiant devices. The temperatures achieved ranged between 40 and 43°C and were maintained for 1 to 5 hours.

The antineoplastic drugs combined with hyperthermia were cisplatin, BCNU, etoposide, cyclophosphamide, DX, and interferon, usually administered as soon as the target temperature was reached.

Thus far, a total of 36 patients have been treated by different investigators, with systemic thermochemotherapy. Complete responses have been observed in three patients (8.8%), and partial responses in eight (23.5%), with responses lasting from 2 to 12 months. Gerard et al. [70] reported the highest percentage of long-term responders (Table 11).

Discussion

There is substantial in vitro, in vivo, and clinical evidence demonstrating the clear antineoplastic activity of hyperthermia, especially when combined with chemotherapy. The greater efficacy of the combined treatment is based on some pharmacokinetic and pharmacodynamic modifications induced by hyperthermia. These involve a greater concentration of the drug within the tumor and a greater efficacy with regard to cellular targets such as DNA [28]. In addition, the ability of hyperthermia to inhibit sublethal damage from chemotherapy should be emphasized [38].

The combination of hyperthermia and chemotherapy has been used for treating soft tissue sarcomas that are often aggressive and show subclinical loco-regional spreading before systemic dissemination [71,72].

In theory, H.A.P. appears to be tailored for the treatment of these tumors for several reasons: (1) the perfusional treatment involves the entire tumor-bearing limb, with possible control of metastatic foci; (2) much higher concentrations of antineoplastic drugs can be given through the perfusional circuit, providing a greater tumor uptake [63]; (3) the high temperatures and the drugs potentiate each other's activity; and (4) the tumor mass shrinkage after H.A.P. permits conservative rather than demolitive surgery.

We have treated 70 patients in different protocols in an attempt to improve regional disease control and augment the possibility of carrying out limb-sparing surgery, while also evaluating the impact on long-term cure.

The results obtained should be interpreted in the light of the characteristics of the patients treated: 48 out of 70 (65.5%) had Stage III—IVA disease, and 38 (54.3%) were recurrent after surgery, radiotherapy, and/or chemotherapy.

Surgery and radiotherapy can reduce blood flow and drug uptake by causing vascular sclerosis, while tumors previously treated with chemotherapy become less responsive to further treatments.

In terms of overall survival, there is a statistically significant difference between patients with primary or recurrent tumors (Table 7). This was confirmed in a multivariate analysis where the number of previous relapses, together with the tumor extension and type of protocol adopted, showed independent values as survival predictors (Table 8).

The protocol including radiotherapy before tumor removal provided better loco-regional control and a higher rate of conservative surgery without limb functionality impairment (Tables 5 and 6). Lethi et al. and Stehlin et al. have reported similar findings. We may therefore hypothesize that the potential efficacy in tumor control could be even greater by using drugs with higher efficacy against soft tissue sarcomas, than by using L-PAM and DACT, which have shown a poor activity when employed as single agents [73-75]. Doxorubicin could be the antineoplastic drug of choice, given its well-documented tumor-specific activity and its synergism with heat [76].

In a phase I study, we employed escalating doses of DX (1, 1.2, 1.4, and 1.6 mg/kg of b.w.) during the perfusion. The maximum tolerable dose was 1.4 mg/kg b.w., with temperatures never exceeding 41.8°C.

The development of technically advanced devices has permitted carrying out the loco-regional hyperthermic treatment of superficial and deep-seated tumors with nonionizing energies. There is still difficulty in reaching high

142

and homogeneous temperatures and in reliably monitoring the heating during the treatment of deep-seated tumors.

Preliminary results reported by Jabboury and Issels, however, seem promising; objective response rates of 50% and 64%, respectively, have been obtained in patients who failed after conventional treatment. These data are consistent wth those reported by Storm et al., who obtained objective responses by combining hyperthermia with the same drugs that had been ineffective when normothermically applied.

Objective responses have been obtained in all the studies employing high temperatures, while stable lesions were observed in studies employing low average temperatures, which emphasizes the importance of reaching the highest possible temperature (Table 9).

Few pilot studies have been conducted on the clinical application of systemic hyperthermia and chemotherapy. Two main limitations hamper the potential effectiveness of these two modalities when systemically applied: the level of hyperthermia and the drug dosage. In fact, the temperature can usually not exceed 42°C to avoid cardiovascular and cerebral complications. On the other hand, the relatively low temperatures applied cannot be compensated by high drug dosages because their systemic administration could be fatal for the patients.

However, complete and partial responses (11 out of 13) have been reported by Bull et al. [11] and Gerard et al. [69] in previously treated patients, although the responses were not long lasting.

In terms of cost benefit, it is difficult to assess the effectiveness of systemic thermochemotherapy for the treatment of metastatic soft tissue sarcomas. Further studies in selected patients and in experienced centers are warranted.

In conclusion, thermochemotherapy has proven to be effective in the treatment of soft tissue sarcoma. Regardless of the hyperthermic treatment employed, the combined treatment has provided objective responses in patients who had failed after conventional treatments. The hyperthermia level is crucial for the tumor response. Drugs able to modify the tumor blood flow represent a new tool in hyperthermic treatments, given their ability to selectively increase the tumor temperature.

Acknowledgments

This work was partially supported by grants from the Italian Ministry of Health, Special Project "Hyperthermia", and the A.I.R.C.

References

1. Busch W: Uber den einfluss welchen heftiger erysipelen zuweilen auf organisierte Neubildungen aushen. Verhandlungen des Naturhistorischer. Vereins Preussicher Rheinalds Westphalen 23:28—30, 1866.

2. Coley WB: The treatment of malignant tumors by repeated inoculations of erysipelas with a report of original cases. Ann J Med Sci 105:487—511, 1893.
3. Rohdenburg GL et al.: The effect of combined radiation and heat on neoplasms. Arch Surg 2:1548—1554, 1906.
4. Warren SL: Preliminary study on the effect of artificial fever upon hopeless tumor cases. AJR 33:75—87, 1935.
5. Cavaliere R et al.: Selective heat sensitivity of cancer cells: Biochemical an clinical studies. Cancer 20:1351—1381, 1967.
6. Hunt JW: Applications of microwaves, ultrasounds and radio frequencies heating in vivo. In: Proceedings of the Third International Symposium on Cancer Therapy by Hyperthermia, Drugs and Radiation. Dethlefsen LA, Dewey WC (eds). Bethesda, MD: pp 447—456, 1984.
7. Weisser M et al.: Advanced technique in localized current field hyperthermia. Recent Results Cancer Res 107:87—92, 1988.
8. Gerner EW: Thermotolerance. In: Hyperthermia in cancer therapy. Storm FK (ed). Boston: GK Hall, pp 141—162, 1983.
9. Field SB et al.: Thermotolerance: A review of observations and possible mechanisms. Natl Cancer Inst Monogr 61:193—201, 1982.
10. Cavaliere R et al.: Regional perfusion hyperthermia. In: Hyperthermia in cancer therapy. Storm FK (ed). Boston: GK Hall, pp 369—399, 1983.
11. Bull JMC: An update on anticancer effects of a combination of chemotherapy and hyperthermia. Cancer Res 44 (Suppl):4853—4856, 1984.
12. Bicher HI et al.: Clinical thermoradiotherapy. In: Hyperthermia in cancer therapy. Storm FK (ed). Boston: GK Hall, 1987.
13. Overgaard J: Combined hyperthermia and radiation treatment of malignant melanoma. In: Hyperthermic oncology 1988. Sugohare T, Saito M (eds). London: Taylor–Francis, pp 464—468, 1988.
14. Arcangeli G: Analysis of results in neck node metastases from tumors of the head and neck. Recent Results Cancer Res 107:118—122, 1988.
15. Hahn GM: Hyperthermia and cancer. New York: Plenum, pp 74—85, 1982.
16. Hahn GM et al.: Thermochemotherapy: Synergism between hyperthermia (42—43 C°) and adriamycin (or bleomycin) in mammalian cell inactivation. Proc Natl Acad Sci USA 12:937—940, 1975.
17. Hahn GM: Potential for therapy of drugs and hyperthermia. Cancer Res 39:2264—2268, 1979.
18. Moricca G et al.: Hyperthermic treatment of tumors: Experimental and clinical applications. Recent Results Cancer Res 59:112—151, 1977.
19. Li GC et al.: Correlation between synthesis of heat shock proteins and development of thermoresistence in Chinese hamster fibroblasts. Proc Natl Acad Sci USA 79:3219—3222, 1982.
20. Tomasovic SP et al.: Heat stress proteins and thermal resistence in rat mammary tumor cells. Radiat Res 70:610—611, 1977.
21. Reinhold HS et al.: Enhancement of thermal damage to sandwich tumors by additional treatment. In: Proceedings of the First Meeting of the European Group on Hyperthermia in Radiation Oncology, Arcangeli G, Mauro F (eds). Milan: Masson, pp 179—183, 1980.
22. Kim JH et al.: Lonidamine: A hyperthermic sensitizer of HeLa cells in culture and of Meth-A tumor in vivo. Oncology 41 (Suppl 1):30—35, 1984.
23. Kim JH et al.: Quercitin, an inhibitor of lactate transport and hyperthermic sensitizer of HeLa cells. Cancer Res 44:1165—1168, 1980.
24. Barlogie B et al.: In vitro thermochemotherapy of human colon cancer cells with CDDP and mytomicin C. Cancer Res 40:1165—1162, 1980.
25. Herman TS: Effect of temperature on the cytotoxicity of vindesine, amsacrine and mitoxantrone. Cancer Treat Rep 67:1019—1022, 1983.

26. Johnson HA et al.: Thermal enhancement of thiotepa cytotoxicity. J Natl Cancer Inst 50:903—908, 1973.
27. Jirtle RL: Chemical modification of tumor blood flow. Int J Hyperthermia 4:355—372, 1988.
28. Dahl O: Interaction of hyperthermia and chemotherapy. Recent Results Cancer Res 107:157—169, 1988.
29. Teicher BA et al.: Enhancement by hyperthermia of the in vitro cytotoxicity of mytomicin C toward hypoxic tumor cells. Cancer Res 41:1096—1099, 1981.
30. Clawson RE et al.: Hyperthermic modification of cyclophosphamide metabolism in rat hepatic microsomes and liver slices. Life Sci 28:1133—1137, 1981.
31. Wallner KE et al.: Hyperthermic potentiation of cis-diammine dichloroplatinum (II) cytotoxicity in Chinese hamster ovary cells resistant to the drug. Cancer Res 46:6242—6245, 1986.
32. Alberts DS et al.: Therapeutic synergism of hyperthermia-cis-platinum in a mouse tumor model. J Natl Cancer Inst 65:455—461, 1980.
33. Meyn RE et al.: Thermal enhancement of DNA strand breakage in mammalian cells treatment with bleomycin. Int J Radiat Oncol Biol Phys 5:1487—1489, 1979.
34. Kubota Y et al.: Effect of hyperthermia on DNA single strand breaks induced by bleomycin in HeLa cells. Gann 70:681—685, 1979.
35. Smith PJ et al.: Interaction between bleomycin, hyperthermia and calmodulin inhibitor (trifluoperazine) in mouse tumor cells. II. DNA damage, repair and chromatin changes. Br J Cancer 53:105—114, 1986.
36. Djordjevic O et al.: The combined effects of hyperthermia and a chemotherapeutic agent on DNA in isolated mammalian cells. In: Cancer therapy by hyperthermia and radiation. Streffer C et al. (eds). Munich: Urban and Schwarzenberg, pp 278—280, 1978.
37. Johnson HA et al.: Thermal enhancement of thio-tepa cytotoxicity. J Natl Cancer Inst 50:903—908, 1973.
38. Spiro IJ et al.: Effect of hyperthermia on CHO DNA polymerase alfa and beta. Radiation Res 89:134—149, 1982.
39. Arrick BA, Nathan CF: Glutathione metabolism as a determinant of therapeutic efficacy: A review. Cancer Res 44:4224—4232, 1984.
40. Shrieve DC et al.: Cellular glutathione, thermal sensitivity and thermotolerance in Chinese hamster fibroblasts and their heat-resistant variants. Cancer Res 46:1684—1687, 1986.
41. Joiner MC et al.: Response of two mouse tumors to hyperthermia with CCNU or melphalan. Br J Cancer 45:19—26, 1982.
42. Leeds DE et al.: Internal organ hypoxia during hyperthermic cancer therapy in humans. Proceedings of the Third International Symposium on Cancer Therapy by Hyperthermic Drugs and Radiation, Fort Collins, CO, p 3, 1980.
43. Bleehn NM et al.: Interaction of hyperthermia and the hypoxic cells sensitizer. RO-07-0582 in the EMT6 mouse tumor. Br J Cancer 35:299—306, 1977.
44. Kapp DS et al.: Thermosensitization by sulphydril compounds of exponentially growing Chinese hamster cells. Cancer Res 29:4630—4635, 1977.
45. Robins IH et al.: Systemic lidocaine enhancement of hyperthermia-induced tumor regression in transplantable murine tumor models. Cancer Res 43:3187—3191, 1983.
46. Herman TS et al.: Reversal of resistance to metothrexate hyperthermia in Chinese hamster ovary cells. Cancer Res 41:3840—3843, 1981.
47. Marmor JE: Interaction of hyperthermia and chemotherapy on animals. Cancer Res 89:2269—2276, 1979.
48. Minmaugh EG et al.: Effect of W.B.H. on the deposition and metabolism of ADR in rabbits. Cancer Res 38:1420—1425, 1978.
49. Kuori M et al.: Antitumor effect of interferon combined with hyperthermia against experimental brain tumor. Proceedings of the Fifth International Symposium of Hyperthermia Oncology, Kyoto, Japan, Aug 29—Sept 3, 1988, pp 232—233.

50. Kallinowski F et al.: Effect of tumor necrosis factor alpha on tumor blood flow and hyperthermic treatment. Oncologie 12:131—135, 1989.
51. Maeta M et al.: The effect of angiotensin II on blood flow in tumors during localized hyperthermia. Int J Hyperthermia 5:191—197, 1989.
52. Yamanchi N et al.: Antitumor synergism of recombinant human tumor necrosis factors and hyperthermia. Proceedings of the Fifth International Symposium of Hyperthermia Oncology, Kyoto, Japan, Aug 29—Sept 3, 1988, pp 282—284.
53. Yasue S et al.: On combination therapy of selective local hyperthermia and local immunomodulator. Proceedings of the Fifth International Symposium of Hyperthermia Oncology, Kyoto, Japan, Aug 29—Sept 3, 1988, pp 234—235.
54. Greco C et al.: Effect of sequential hyperthermia and chemotherapy on the survival of a thermoresistant human melanoma cell line. Cancer Biochem Biophys 9:223—232, 1987.
55. Di Filippo F et al.: Prognostic variables in recurrent limb melanoma treated with hyperthermia antiblastic perfusion. Cancer 63:2551—2561, 1989.
56. Marijnissen H et al: Interstitial photodynamic therapy of rat rhabdomyosarcoma: Dose effect relationships. Seventh Annual Meeting of the European Society for Therapeutic Radiology and Oncology, Den Haag, The Netherlands, September 5—8, 1988, p 391.
57. Pfeffer HR et al.: Platinum distribution, retention and DNA cross-linking in tumors and normal tissue of mice treated with CDDP and local hyperthermia. Thirty-Seventh Annual Meeting of the Radiation Research Society and Ninth Annual Meeting of the North American Hyperthermia Group. March 18—23, 1989, Seattle, WA, p 27, 1989.
58. Nishiue T et al.: Studies on combination of hyperthermia and chemotherapy for cancer. Proceedings of the Fifth International Symposium of Hyperthermia Oncology, Kyoto, Japan, Aug 29—Sept 3, 1988.
59. George C et al.: Enhancement of hyperthermic response of a mouse fibrosarcoma by membrane specific drugs. Proceedings of the Fifth International Symposium of Hyperthermia Oncology Kyoto, Japan, Aug 29—Sept 3, 1988.
60. Baba H et al.: Effect of whole body hyperthermia combined with adriamycin on tumor and normal tissue in rats. Thirty-Seventh Annual Meeting of the Radiation Research Society and Ninth Annual Meeting of the North American Hyperthermia Group, March 18—23, 1989, Seattle, WA, p 34, 1989.
61. Milligan AJ: Whole body hyperthermia induction techniques. Cancer Res 44 (Suppl): 4869—4872, 1984.
62. Di Filippo F et al.: Role of hyperthermic perfusion as a first step in the treatment of soft tissue sarcoma of the extremities. World J Surg 12:332—339, 1982.
63. Di Filippo F et al.: Hyperthermic perfusion with cisplatin: Standardization of treatment parameters. Regional Cancer Treat 2:131—136, 1989.
64. Lehti PM et al.: Improved survival for soft tissue sarcoma of the extremities by regional hyperthermic perfusion, local excision and radiation therapy. Surg Gynecol Obstet 162: 142—152, 1986.
65. Stehlin JS et al.: 15-Year experience with hyperthermic perfusion for treatment of soft tissue sarcoma and malignant melanoma of the extremities. In: Hyperthermia and radiation therapy/chemotherapy in the treatment of cancer. Vaeth JM (ed). San Francisco: pp 177—182, 1984.
66. Jabboury K et al.: Local hyperthermia for resistant soft tissue sarcoma. Thirty-Fourth Annual Meeting of the Radiation Research Society, Las Vegas, April 1986, p 18.
67. Issels R et al.: Regional hyperthermia combined with systemic chemotherapy. Fourth Internation Conference on Advances in Regional Cancer Therapy, June 5—7, 1989, Berchtessgaden, 1989.
68. Cavaliere R: Unpublished data.
69. Storm FK et al.: Magnetic induction hyperthermia: Results of a five-year multiinstitutional national cooperative trial in advanced cancer patients. Cancer 55:2677—2687, 1985.
70. Gerard H et al.: Doxorubicin, cyclophosphamide and WBH for treatment of advanced soft tissue sarcomas. Cancer 53:2585—2591, 1984.

71. Cantin J et al.: The problem of local recurrence after treatment of soft tissue sarcoma. Ann Surg 168:47—53, 1968.
72. Heise HW et al.: Recurrence-free survival time for surgically treated soft tissue sarcoma patients: Multivariate analysis of five prognostic factors. Cancer 57:172—177, 1986.
73. Cruz AB et al.: Combination chemotherapy for soft tissue sarcoma: A phase II study. J Surg Oncol II:313—323, 1979.
74. Greenhall MS et al.: Chemotherapy for soft tissue sarcoma. Surg Gynecol Obstet 162:193—198, 1986.
75. Verweij J, Pinedo HM: Chemotherapy in advanced soft tissue sarcoma. In: Clinical management of soft tissue sarcoma Pinedo HM, Verweij J (eds). Boston: Martinus Nijhoff, pp 81—88, 1986.
76. Chang AE et al.: Sarcomas of the soft tissue. In: Cancer: Principles and practice of oncology. De Vita VT, Hellman S, Rosenberg SA (eds). Philadelphia: JB Lippincott, pp 1345—1398, 1989.
77. Rosenberg SA: Prospective randomized trials demonstrating the efficacy of adjuvant chemotherapy in adults with soft tissue sarcomas of the extremities. Cancer 52:424—434, 1983.
78. Gherlinzoni F et al.: A randomized trial for the treatment of high-grade soft tissue sarcomas of the extremities: Preliminary observations. J Clin Oncol 4:552—558, 1986.

11. Soft Tissue Sarcomas of Children

Charles B. Pratt and Larry E. Kun

Introduction

Soft tissue sarcomas have been defined as malignant tumors involving non-epithelial extraskeletal tissues of the body, exclusive of the reticuloendothelial system, glia, and supporting tissues of various parenchymal organs [1]. The soft tissues are represented by voluntary muscles, fat, and fibrous tissue, along with the vessels servicing these tissues [1]. By convention, the soft tissues include the peripheral nervous system because tumors arising from nerves present as soft tissue masses and pose similar problems in differential diagnosis and therapy [1]. Embryologically, the soft tissues are derived principally from mesoderm, with some contribution for ectoderm [1].

For adults there has been a change in the relative incidence of various soft tissue sarcomas, varying with the time of reports from 1962 to the present [1]. As larger series of soft tissue sarcomas, other than rhabdomyosarcoma (RMS), are reported, it is expected that reclassification by soft tissue pathologists will emphasize an evolution and shifting of histologic classifications. Reviews of specimens by panels and pathologists indicate discrepancies in pathologic interpretation of diagnosis [2], as well as in grade of tumor [3].

Despite variations in histology, soft tissue tumors of children behave in similar ways characterized by (1) pseudoencapsulation by surrounding fibrous and reactive connective tissue, with tumor infiltration beyond the pseudocapsule; (2) spread along musculoaponeurotic planes; and (3) distant spread via hematogenous routes, with lymphatic spread being relatively rare [4-11].

Classification of pediatric soft tissue sarcomas has changed over the past 30 years such that larger percentages are now classified as RMS (65 to 70%), and smaller percentages are considered to be unclassified (5 to 10%) [7].

Prognostic factors involved with pediatric soft tissue sarcomas include the tumor size, tumor location, extent of tumor (stage or grouping), histologic cell type, and pathologic grade [7].

Soft tissue sarcomas of children may develop at any site [1,4,7], usually

Pinedo, H.M., Verweij, J., and H.D. Suit (eds.): Soft Tissue Sarcomas: New Developments in the Multidisciplinary Approach to Treatment. © *1991 Kluwer Academic Publishers, Boston. ISBN: 0–7923–1139–6. All rights reserved.*

presenting as a mass with or without pain. The mass is usually discovered by the child or his parent. The mass may be small if it is located in a subcutaneous region. Masses that involve the extremity, retroperitoneal, or intrathoracic areas may become extremely large before discovery.

The symptoms produced by these cancers are related to tumor growth or pressure on adjacent structures, or to hemorrhage, obstruction, or perforation of viscera, or necrosis of these tumors. Sarcomas usually are painless, but pain may develop acutely after spontaneous hemorrhage or after trauma. Patients often date symptoms to an injury that has no relationship to the development of the sarcoma. Tumor necrosis is associated with the insidious onset of pain or the direct compression of nerves or neurovascular bundle. A schwannoma or neurogenic sarcoma arising in a peripheral nerve may cause pain within the distribution of that nerve.

Cranial nerve dysfunction may occur in patients with soft tissue sarcomas involving the head and neck region. Intrathoracic sarcomas can produce shortness of breath and may be associated with pleural effusion. Retroperitoneal disease generally presents as a large mass that is discovered as incidental abdominal enlargement. Symptoms of gastrointestinal or urinary tract obstruction may occur. Soft tissue sarcomas of the extremity can disturb function of the limb, but are associated with pain only if there is direct bony or neurovascular involvement by the tumor.

Bone marrow metastases occur in about 10% of RMS cases, but are rare in the other soft tissue sarcomas. Direct invasion of bone occurs most often in RMS arising in the head and neck region, most typically in parameningeal sites (e.g., nasopharyngeal, paranasal sinuses, middle ear); it is rare to see bone invasion in other histologic types [8]. Lymph node metastasis is uncommon in nonrhabdomyosarcomatous soft tissue sarcoma (NRSTS) [11]. In RMS, lymph node metastasis is apparent in 5 to 40% of the cases: more commonly in lesions arising in the genitourinary tract [12,13].

Childhood sarcomas rarely are associated with paraneoplastic syndromes [14]. Hypoglycemia has accompanied advanced fibrosarcoma, schwannoma, and hemangiopericytoma; the hypoglycemia associated with hemangiopericytoma may be produced by substances with nonsuppressive insulin-like activity.

High-grade sarcomas occasionally produce fever, which may be associated with tumor necrosis.

For soft tissue sarcomas of children, the grouping system of the Intergroup Rhabdomyosarcoma Study Committee has achieved almost universal use because of its relevance to pediatric sarcomas. Alternative use of the TNM system is yet undergoing evaluation for RMS [15]. By convention, sarcomas of the brain and liver are excluded from the NRSTS, and additional discussion focuses on the more common tumors, other than RMS, involving the head, neck, trunk, and extremities. Although different in origin, a description of primitive neuroectodermal tumors is included.

150

Table 1. Nonrhabdomyosarcoma soft tissue sarcomas, St. Jude Children's Research Hospital, 1962—1988: Patient distribution by site and clinical grouping.

Site	Clinical groupings				All groups
	I	II	III	IV	
Head and neck	6 (30)*	4 (20)	8 (40)	2 (10)	20 (13.9)
Trunk	20 (29)	9 (13)	23 (33)	17 (25)	69 (48.3)
Extremity	31 (57)	8 (15)	6 (11)	9 (17)	54 (37.8)
All sites	57 (40)	21 (15)	37 (26)	28 (19)	143 (100)

* Number of patients (%) in each group according to site of malignancy. Percentages for all sites and all groups are based on the total number (143) of patients in this study.

Incidence

RMS and the other soft tissue sarcomas of children comprise about 10% of all tumors seen in childhood and adolesence [16]. RMS has been extensively reviewed both in the European literature [13,17-19] and in the U.S. [20-23]. Site-specific presentations have been outlined for the more common regions of origin in the head and neck, genitourinary tract, extremities, and trunk. The NRSTS represent 25 to 35% of all soft tissue sarcomas occurring in patients younger than 20 years [1,7]. Because of their rarity and diverse characteristics, information about the frequency of these tumors or their sites of origin is limited. Therefore, we reviewed the 143 patients with NRSTS seen at St. Jude Children's Research Hospital during a 27-year period to January 1989. These 143 cases represent 25% of the 573 patients with soft tissues sarcomas seen during that period.

In Table 1, NRSTS are distributed by site and clinical grouping, using the Intergroup Rhabdomyosarcoma Study Committee scheme. The greatest number of the NRSTS occur in the trunk, representing 48% of the total patients. By clinical grouping, 40% of all patients had group I disease, 15% had clinical group II disease, 26% had clinical group III disease, and 19% had clinical group IV disease.

Survival by histologic type and clinical grouping for patients with NRSTS of the head and neck region is depicted in Table 2. These rare soft tissue sarcomas represent a mixture of histologic types, the most frequent of which is schwannoma. Survival has been good for patients who had localized tumors that were resectable or those with microscopic residual tumor.

Survival by clinical grouping of patients with NRSTS of the trunk is shown in Table 3. This was the most common tumor site in this series. Survival was good for individuals with resectable disease, even in a location associated with an unfavorable outcome in RMS. For the trunk area, the most frequently encountered soft tissue NRSTS were primitive neuroectodermal tumors, schwannomas, and extraosseous Ewing sarcoma.

Table 2. Nonrhabdomyosarcoma soft tissue sarcoma of head and neck, St. Jude Children's Research Hospital, 1962—1988: Survival by clinical grouping.

Tumor	Clinical groupings (number surviving/treated)			
	I	II	III	IV
Synovial sarcoma			0/1	
Fibrosarcoma, infantile	0/1			0/1
Fibrosarcoma	1/1			
Malignant fibrous histiocytoma			0/1	
Epithelioid sarcoma	1/1			
Schwannoma	0/1	1/1	0/3	
Alveolar soft part sarcoma	1/1			
Myeloid chondrosarcoma	1/1			
Sarcoma, not otherwise specified			1/1	0/1
Hemangiopericytoma		2/2	0/1	
Hemangioendothelioma		0/1*	1/1	
Total patients	4/6	3/4	2/8	0/2

* Died of accidental causes.

Table 3. Nonrhabdomyosarcoma soft tissue sarcoma of the trunk, St. Jude Children's Research Hospital, 1962—1988: Survival by clinical grouping.

Tumor	Clinical groupings (number surviving/treated)			
	I	II	III	IV
Synovial sarcoma	2/3		0/1	0/2
Fibrosarcoma, infantile	1/1	1/1		
Fibrosarcoma	2/2		0/1*	
Malignant fibrous histiocytoma	2/2	1/1		0/1
Epithelioid sarcoma				0/1
Schwannoma	1/1	0/1	0/3	0/3
Alveolar soft part sarcoma	2/2		1/1	
Sarcoma, not otherwise specified	2/2		0/2	1/1
Leiomyosarcoma	0/2	1/2		0/2
Angiosarcoma			0/1	
Liposarcoma	1/1		1/2	0/1
Mesothelioma			1/1	
Extraosseous Ewing sarcoma	2/8			
Primitive neuroectodermal tumor	1/1	4/4	2/11	1/6
Total patients	16/20	7/9	5/23	2/17

The second most frequent site of NRSTS was in the extremities. The most common tumor type was synovial sarcoma. Survival (Table 4) was related to the clinical grouping and was better for individuals with clinical groups I or II disease than for clinical groups III or IV disease.

Table 5 combines Tables 2 through 4 and indicates survival by clinical grouping of patients with tumors at all sites. There was no statistically significant difference in survival by histologic type.

Table 4. Nonrhabdomyosarcoma soft tissue sarcoma of the extremities, St. Jude Children's Research Hospital, 1962—1988: Survival by clinical grouping.

Tumor	Clinical groupings (number surviving/treated)			
	I	II	III	IV
Synovial sarcoma	13/16	2/2	0/3	1/4*
Fibrosarcoma, infantile	2/3			
Fibrosarcoma	1/1			
Malignant fibrous histiocytoma	4/4			0/2
Epithelioid sarcoma	0/1			
Schwannoma	1/1	1/2		
Alveolar soft part sarcoma	0/1			
Myxoid chondrosarcoma				0/1
Sarcoma, not otherwise specified	1/1	1/1		
Hemangiopericytoma	1/1		0/1	0/1
Angiosarcoma			0/1	
Liposarcoma			0/1	
Dermatofibrosarcoma protuberans	1/1	1/1		
Extraosseous Ewing sarcoma	0/1			
Primitive neuroectodermal tumor		1/2		0/1
Total patients	24/31	6/8	0/6	1/9

* Living with disease. Died in accidental causes.

Table 5. Nonrhabdomyosarcoma soft tissue sarcoma at all sites: Survival by clinical grouping.

Tumor	Clinical groupings (number surviving/treated)				All groups
	I	II	III	IV	
synovial sarcoma	15/19	2/2	0/5	1/6	18/32
Schwannoma	2/3	2/4	0/6	0/3	4/16
Malignant fibrous histiocytoma	6/6	1/1	0/1	0/3	7/11
Fibrosarcoma, infantile	3/5	1/1		0/1	4/7
Fibrosarcoma	4/4		0/1		4/5
Alveolar soft part	3/4*		1/1		4/5
Myxoid chondrosarcoma	1/1			0/1	1/2
Epithelioid sarcoma	1/2			0/1	1/3
Sarcoma, not otherwise specified	3/3	1/1	1/3	1/2	6/9
Hemangiopericytoma	1/1	2/2	0/2	0/1	3/6
Leiomyosarcoma	0/2	1/2		0/2	1/6
Angiosarcoma			0/2		0/2
Liposarcoma	1/1		1/3	0/1	2/5
Dermatofibrosarcoma protuberans	1/1	1/1			2/2
Mesothelioma			1/1		1/1
Hemangioendothelioma		0/1*	1/1		1/2
Extraosseous Ewing sarcoma	3/5				3/5
Primitive neuroectodermal tumor	1/1	5/6	2/11	1/7	9/25
Total patients	45/58	16/21	7/37	3/28	71/143

* One died of accidental causes.

153

The management of patients with RMS has been extensively reported. Evolution to multimodality therapy, using combinations of surgery, irradiation, and chemotherapy, has resulted in high rates of disease control for most early and intermediate stage lesions [7,20-29]. Current research efforts seek to improve local/regional control for tumors that are unresectable due to disease extent and/or site, and to coordinate maximal preservation of function with improved disease control [27].

Management

Patients with NRSTS underwent various surgical techniques for biopsy or resection of the tumor, and many received chemotherapy and/or radiotherapy. Details of these procedures have been published in part by Horowitz et al. [8]. More recently, children have been treated by the Pediatric Oncology Group Protocol 8653/54, entitled "A Study of Childhood Soft Tissue Sarcomas Other Than Rhabdomyosarcoma and its Variants," in which patients receive follow-up evaluation with or without chemotherapy and/or radiotherapy following diagnosis (figure 1).

The approach to the management of the NRSTS of children and adolescents [28-31] in many ways is similar to that for tumors with similar histologies involving adults, for which there is greater experience in management [9,10,32-36]. The preoperative evaluation assesses the local spread and location of distant metastases. Tumors are evaluated by size and frequency and for possible lymph node and distant metastases and for potential resectability [9,10].

Few studies of pediatric sarcomas have indicated the success of local control with surgery alone, radiation therapy alone, or surgery and radiotherapy, in comparison to several studies of similar tumors involving adults. Dose response following radiotherapy for RMS has been addressed in each of the protocols of the Intergroup Rhabdomyosarcoma Study [22-23]. The impact of multiagent chemotherapy has been addressed by Flamant and colleagues at the Institut Gustave Roussy, based upon results obtained before and after 1972 [17], by Voute in the Netherlands [18], and recently by Maurer in the U.S. summarizing the results of treatment in Intergroup Rhabdomyosarcoma Studies I—III [23]. Improved results with regard to complete remission rates (figure 2), survival for clinical group III patients (figure 3), and overall survival have been noted in the successive studies (figure 4) [23].

Surgery

Surgical procedures for soft tissue sarcomas of any type may include fine needle aspiration, needle biopsy, excisional biopsy, incisional biopsy with or without frozen section, or total resection [9,10]. The exact nature of the

154

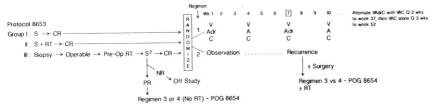

Soft Tissue Sarcoma Study Scheme (POG 8653/8654)

Figure 1. Nonrhabdomyosarcoma soft tissue sarcoma of the Pediatric Oncology Group (POG 8653/8654). Footnotes: V = Vincristine 1.5 mg/m^2 IV (no dose to exceed 2 mg); Adr = Doxorubicin 60 mg/m^2 IV (cumulative dose = 360 mg/m^2; C = Cyclophosphamide 750 mg/m^2 IV; A = Actinomycin D (Dactinomycin) 1.25 mg/m^2 IV (no top dose); DTIC = Imidazole carboxamide 500 mg/m^2 (no top dose); S = Surgery; S^2 = Second surgery 6—12 weeks after completion of radiotherapy; = Evaluation for response and/or recurrence; O = Omit cyclophosphamide if bladder is in field of radiotherapy.

COMPLETE REMISSION DURATION
BY IRS STUDY

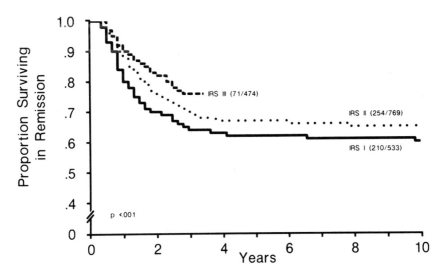

Figure 2. Complete remission rates, Integroup Rhabdomyosarcoma Study protocols I—III [23]. (Figure provided by courtesy of H.M. Maurer, M.D.)

surgical procedure is influenced by the site and the potential resectability of the lesion, in addition to the efficacy of alternating treatments, the latter primarily in RMS. Local control may be more difficult to achieve in the retroperitoneal area or the head and neck area due to the inability to widely excise tumors in these sites. For extremity tumors, local control may be more difficult to obtain in proximal presentation.

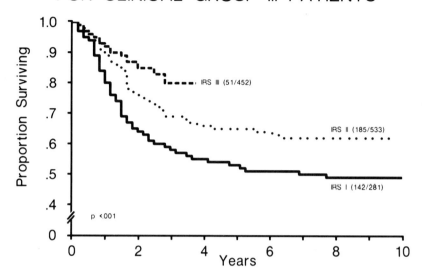

Figure 3. Survival, all patients, Intergroup Rhabdomyosarcoma Study protocols I—III [23]. (Figure provided by courtesy of H.M. Maurer, M.D.)

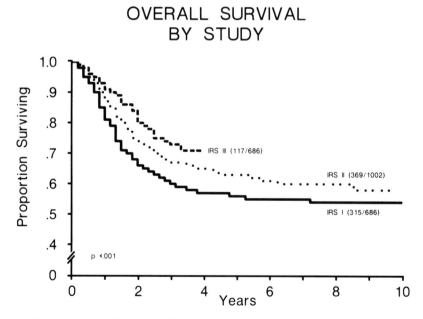

Figure 4. Overall survival, Intergroup Rhabdomyosarcoma Study by successive protocols I—III [23]. (Figure provided by courtesy of H.M. Maurer, M.D.)

For extremity lesions, appropriate surgical procedures have been identified as intracapsular resection, marginal resection, wide resection, radical resection, muscle compartment excisions, or other limb-sparing procedures [4,5]. Amputation may be utilized depending upon the site and extent of the primary tumor and the natural history, primarily for specific types of NRSTS.

Surgery is the primary treatment for NRSTS, which may also require multimodality approaches, including the possible use of chemotherapy and radiation therapy [27,28,30-37]. The shelling out of a lesion is inadequate therapy, allowing local recurrence in as many as 90% of the affected individuals. Wide local excision yields a local recurrence rate of about 50% [37,38]. Local recurrence may be reduced by postoperative radiation therapy after conservative surgical procedures. High local failure rates and high overall failure rates for adult NRSTS range from 38 to 80%, which indicate the need to identify effective adjuvant chemotherapy for adults and children [8,9].

Whether there is a difference in disease-free or overall survival rates [39-43] between patients requiring amputation and those having limb-sparing procedures [44] or local surgical procedures followed by radiation and chemotherapy is not known.

Radiation Therapy

RMS is relatively sensitive to radiation therapy, but requires relatively high total dose to large fields to effect maximal tumor control [7,17,24,25]. In orbital and parameningeal head and neck sites, primary irradiation is highly effective in ensuring disease control. In other sites, coordinated radiation therapy and chemotherapy may result in local/regional control, with limited and tissue-preserving surgery.

Objective responses of NRSTS to radiation therapy have been appreciated for many years. Recommended dosages have been in the range of 60 Gy for adults with microscopic disease [37,45].

Studies are needed of the time-dosage fractionation relationships in children and adults with NRSTS [8-10,34,37,45-47].

Prospective studies of the efficacy of adjuvant irradiation have also been few. Amputation and local surgery with radiotherapy for extremity NRSTS have yielded similar results [8-10]. Studies at our institution [8] were not controlled and failed to demonstrate an advantage for children with NRSTS who received adjuvant chemotherapy with or without irradiation therapy after limited surgery.

By the scheme of the Pediatric Oncology Group Protocols 8653/8654 (figure 1), patients with group I disease receive no radiation therapy. Patients with group II disease receive radiation as primary treatment and then are randomized to receive or to not receive chemotherapy. Patients with groups III and IV tumors receive radiation to the primary tumor site after defining initial response following chemotherapy. Those with group IV disease also receive radiation to the sites of the metastatic tumor.

The volume encompassed by radiation therapy should include the primary tumor area widely, with a 2.5-cm margin beyond the preoperative tumor extent. For groups III and IV, a boost to the initial tumor volume is encouraged, with special consideration for limiting the dosage delivered to growing bones and normal tissues.

Megavoltage equipment is recommended for use with parallel opposed portals (equally, or unevenly weighted), with special attention to normal tissue sparing in extremity lesions. The use of multiple convergent beams or electronbeam therapy may be of value in superficial or chest wall tumors.

Dose relationships for RMS show disease control with microscopic extent at the 40-Gy level [24,25]. For patients with group III RMS, current studies focus on hyperfractionated irradiation (e.g., 60 Gy at 110 cGy twice daily in IRS 4) in an attempt to improve local control without excessive toxicity [29]. For NRSTS, the POG study has recommended a total dose of 45 to 50 Gy for children less than 5 to 6 years old; in older children, wide field irradiation to 45 to 55 Gy is followed by reduced fields to dose levels of 60 to 65 Gy.

Brachytherapy may be utilized for selected tumor sites, primarily in the extremities or peripheral truncal sites [48]. Use of external irradiation combined with brachytherapy to the primary site may be ideal in applicable cases [49,50].

Chemotherapy

The use of specific chemotherapy for NRSTS in children remains ill defined [8]. The value of chemotherapy after resection of localized tumors is controversial because the survival rate for these tumors is greater than 75%. To qualify as a candidate for adjuvant chemotherapy, the patient's tumor must have great potential to metastasize and have a high mortality rate associated with metastases. The tumor must be one for which there is a reasonable possibility of response to chemotherapy.

Phase I and II chemotherapy trials since 1960 have contributed to the present multiagent chemotherapy schemes for the various soft tissue sarcomas. These studies have indicated that vincristine [51], cyclophosphamide [52], dactinomycin [53], doxorubicin [54,55], imidazole carboxamide [56], cisplatin [57], etoposide [58], and ifosfamide [59,60], alone or in combination [26,54,61-69], have activity against soft tissue sarcomas. Survival in adults has been influenced by the delivery of these agents in combination. The most effective of these agents probably are vincristine, cyclophosphamide, doxorubicin, ifosfamide, and dactinomycin [51-55,59,60].

Few studies have been instituted to determine the effectiveness of adjuvant chemotherapy for the NRSTS of young patients [8], but important studies are now in progress in Europe [30] and in the U.S. (figure 1) [62].

158

Phase II studies of adults and children helped to demonstrate the effectiveness of single-agent therapy on measurable disease, either primary or metastatic. Multiple drug combinations are being used with and without radiotherapy. Several of these studies are randomized, permitting answers to important epidemiologic questions.

The oncologist who treats these rare pediatric sarcomas at the present time has several options for primary treatment:

1. The Pediatric Oncology Group Protocols 8653/8654 (figure 1) will determine whether adjuvant chemotherapy increases the relapse-free survival rate of patients with localized, completely resected NRSTS with or without postoperative irradiation. Chemotherapeutic agents include vincristine, cyclophosphamide, dactinomycin, doxorubicin with or without imidazole carboxamide (DTIC), for patients with metastatic NRSTS at diagnosis, with previously "untreated" recurrent NRSTS, or with localized, persistent, residual NRSTS after surgery and radiation therapy. Details of the treatment scheme, including dosages of chemotherapeutic agents, are as presented in figure 1.

2. Treatment by the Malignant Mesenchymal Tumor (MMT) Protocol '89 of the Societe Internationale Oncologie Pediatrique (SIOP) [67] uses surgery, radiation, and chemotherapy (ifosfamide 3 gm/m^2 plus Mesna on days 1 and 2, vincristine 1.5 mg/m^2 [maximum 2 mg] IV on days 1 and 14, and dactinomycin 0.9 mg/m^2 [maximum 1 g] on days 1 and 2, with a 14-day interval between courses). Ten courses of chemotherapy are given without radiation if a complete response (proven by surgery) is obtained. If a partial remission is obtained, patients receive two to six courses of cisplatin and adriamycin. If a surgically documented complete response is obtained, treatment is stopped and radiotherapy is not given; if a partial response is obtained, further surgery or radiotherapy become the options.

3. Treatment by the protocol of the Pediatric Branch, National Cancer Institute [62], Bethesda, Maryland, includes vincristine 2 mg/m^2 (maximum dose 2 mg) on day 1, doxorubicin 35 mg/m^2 on days 1 and 2, cyclophosphamide 900 mg/m^2 days 1 and 2 IV over 1 hour with Mesna 360 mg/m^2 IV over 1 hour mixed with cyclophosphamide, and followed by Mesna 120 mg/m^2 as a continuous infusion during hours 2 to 5, and then at hours 5, 8, 11, 14, 17, and 20 IV over 15 to 30 minutes or orally. Vincristine, doxorubicin, and cyclophosphamide are subsequently alternated with ifosfamide 1,800 mg/m^2/day and etoposide 100 mg/m^2/day for 5 days at 3-week intervals. Vincristine is delivered weekly on weeks 0, 1, 2, 4, 5, 6, 12, 24, 30, 36, and 42. Radiation therapy is delivered over 6 to 8 weeks, beginning at week 13; ifosfamide-etoposide-Mesna are given every 3 weeks during radiation therapy. After radiation therapy, dosages of doxorubicin and cyclophosphamide, respectively, are changed to 50 mg/m^2 once and 1200 mg/m^2 once, rather than on consecutive days. In all, 18 cycles of chemotherapy are planned for delivery during 51 weeks. Early positive results of this treatment have been demonstrated [62].

For patients with recurrent disease after earlier responses or for patients who fail to achieve a complete response after surgery, chemotherapy, and radiation therapy, there remain optional chemotherapy regimens if the remaining disease cannot be resected or retreated with irradiation (which may include brachytherapy). These chemotherapy options include the use of (1) ifosfamide-etoposide as advocated by Miser and associates [64] and Kung and associates [68], or (2) cisplatin-etoposide in conventional dosages [26] or in high dosages with granulocyte-macrophage colony-stimulating factor or granulocyte colony-stimulating factor, with or without autologous bone marrow transplantation.

Prognosis

The prognosis for patients treated by the protocols of the IRS are demonstrated in figures 2—4 [22-23]. Other alternatives to the treatment of rhabdomyosarcoma include the present protocols of the International Society of Pediatric Oncology, the French Society of Pediatric Oncology, the Italian Society of Pediatric Oncology, the German Society of Pediatric Oncology, the Pediatric Branch of the National Cancer Institute, St. Jude Children's Research Hospital, Memorial Sloan-Kettering Cancer Centers, and other large independent institutions. The NRSTS of childhood may occur at the same sites as the childhood rhabdomyosarcomas [70-91].

Overall, it can be stated that the prognosis for our patients with NRSTS depends upon the site and clinical grouping, with a better outcome for individuals with groups I or II NRSTS, with survival rates of 77 and 76%, respectively (Table 5). Unfortunately, the exact contribution of surgery, radiation, and chemotherapy to these results cannot be adequately addressed because of the varying treatments and lack of control groups.

NRSTS that occur in adolescents and adults may occur as second malignant neoplasms following earlier treatment with radiation and/or chemotherapy [92]. Four such patients have been treated at our institution, and their tumors are not included within the analysis in Tables 1 through 5. Soft tissue or bony sarcomas only rarely develop following earlier treatment for acute leukemia. Treatment options for these second tumors depend upon the site and resectability of the tumor, and treatment may also be limited by the type and amount of prior chemotherapy and radiotherapy.

A recent report of 53 postirradiation soft tissue sarcomas indicated that these poorly differentiated tumors were detected after a mean latency period of 10 years and that the patients had dismal prognoses [92]. Most of these tumors were malignant fibrous histiocytomas, followed in frequency by extraskeletal osteosarcomas, fibrosarcomas, schwannomas, extraskeletal chondrosarcomas, and angiosarcomas.

Because of the rarity of sarcomas in children and adolescents, patients with these tumors should be admitted to therapeutic protocols that may contribute to the knowledge about the natural history, epidemiology, and therapeutic results. Therapeutic modalities must be tailored for the site and extent of the disease, the patient's age, and the normal tissues that may be affected by the surgical procedures, radiation, and chemotherapy. Tailoring should be performed within the setting of the multimodality protocol chosen for patient. The exact influence that the histology of these rare tumors has on ultimate prognosis remains to be determined.

There remains the need for greater uniformity in pathologic interpretation and reporting, so that frequency and treatment results may be compared. With the various tumors at differing sites, it becomes evident that achieving local control is important, for salvage after failure of local control is difficult to achieve, even with the use of combined modality therapy. Additionally, tumors that cannot be radically resected require radiotherapy to improve the possibility of local control. At the present time, the tumor dose for rhabdomyosarcoma should be >40 Gy, and for the other soft tissue sarcomas should be >50 Gy, by conventional fractionation techniques. The efficacy of chemotherapy for all stages of rhabdomyosarcoma has been demonstrated (figures 2—4). For other soft tissue sarcomas, some evidence of chemotherapy activity is evident, but additional studies are required to define the exact role of chemotherapy in providing ultimate control of these rare tumors.

Acknowledgments

This work was supported in part by Childhood Cancer Program Project Grant CA23099, Cancer Center (CORE) Grant CA21765 from the National Cancer Institute, and by the American Lebanese Syrian Associated Charities (ALSAC). Gratitude is expressed to Mrs. Laural Avery, Mrs. Alvida Cain, Mrs. Debbie Poe, and Miss Patricia Logan for their technical assistance, and to Ms. Linda Wood for typing the manuscript.

References

1. Enzinger FM, Weiss SW: General considerations. In: Soft tissue tumors, 2nd edition. Enzinger FM, Weiss SW (eds). St Louis: CV Mosby, pp 1—18, 1989.
2. Presant CA, Russell WO, Alexander RW, et al.: Soft tissue and bone sarcoma histopathology peer review: The frequency of disagreement in diagnosis and the need for second pathology opinions: The Southeastern Cancer Study Group experience. J Clin Oncol 4:1658—1661, 1986.
3. Coindre JM, Trojani M, Contesso G, et al.: Reproducibility of a histopathologic grading system for adult soft tissue sarcomas. Cancer 58:306—309, 1986.
4. Miser JS, Triche TJ, Pritchard DJ, Kinsella T: Ewing's sarcoma and the nonrhabdomyosarcoma soft tissue sarcomas of childhood. In: Principles and practice of pediatric oncology. Pizzo PA, Poplack DG (eds). Philadelphia: JB Lippincott, pp 678—688, 1989.

5. Simon MA, Enneking WF: The management of soft tissue sarcomas of the extremities. J Bone Joint Surg (Am) 58:317—327, 1976.
6. Weingrad DW, Rosenberg SA: Early lymphatic spread osteogenic and soft tissue sarcomas. Surgery 84:231—240, 1978.
7. Pizzo PA, Horowitz ME, Poplack DG, Hays DM, Kun LE: Solid tumors of childhood. In: Cancer: Principles and practice of oncology, 3rd edition. DeVita VT, Jr, Hillman S, Rosenberg SA (eds). Philadelphia: JB Lippincott, pp 1612—1670, 1989.
8. Horowitz ME, Pratt CB, Webber BL, et al.: Therapy of childhood soft-tissue sarcomas other than rhabdomyosarcoma: A review of 62 cases treated at a single institution. J Clin Oncol 4:559—564, 1986.
9. Chang AE, Rosenberg SA: Clinical evaluation and treatment of soft tissue sarcomas. In: Soft tissue tumors, 2nd edition. Enzinger FM, Weiss SW (eds). St Louis: CV Mosby, pp 19—42, 1988.
10. Chang AE, Rosenberg SA, Glatstein SA, Antman KH: Sarcomas of soft tissues. In: Cancer: Principles and practice of oncology, 3rd edition. DeVita VT, Jr, Hellman S, Rosenberg SA, (eds). Philadelphia: JB Lippincott, pp 1345—1398, 1989.
11. Mazeron JJ, Suit HD: Lymph nodes as sites of metastases from sarcomas of soft tissue. Cancer 60:1800, 1987.
12. Lawrence W, Jr, Hays DM, Heyn R, et al.: Lymphatic metastasis with childhood rhabdomyosarcoma: A report from the Intergroup Rhabdomyosarcoma Study. Cancer 60:910—915, 1987.
13. Kingston JE, McElwain TJ, Malpas JS: Childhood rhabdomyosarcoma: Experience of the Children's Solid Tumor Group. Br J Cancer 48:195—207, 1983.
14. Bunn PA, Jr, Ridgway EC: Paraneoplastic syndromes in cancer. In: Cancer: Principles and practice of oncology, 3rd edition. DeVita VT, Jr, Hellman S, Rosenberg SA (eds). Philadelphia: JB Lippincott, pp 1896—1940, 1989.
15. Lawrence W, Jr, Gehan EA, Hays DM, et al.: Prognostic significance of staging factors of the UICC staging system in childhood rhabdomyosarcoma: A report from the Intergroup Rhabdomyosarcoma Study (IRS-II). J Clin Oncol 5:46—54, 1987.
16. Young JL, Jr, Miller RW: Incidence of malignant tumors in U.S. Children. J Pediatr 86:254, 1975.
17. Flamant F, Hill C: The improvement in survival associated with combined chemotherapy in childhood rhabdomyosarcoma: A historical comparison of 345 patients in the same center. Cancer 53:2417–2421, 1984.
18. Voute PA, Vos A, de Kraker J, et al.: Rhabdomyosarcoma: Chemotherapy and limited supplementary treatment program to avoid mutilation. Natl Cancer Inst Monogr 56:121—125, 1981.
19. Treuner J, Suder J, Gerein V, et al.: Behandlungsergebesse der nichtrabdomyosarcomatösen Weichteilmalegnome im Rahmen der CWI-81-Studie. Klin Pediatr 199:209—217, 1987.
20. Pratt CB, Hustu HO, Kumar APM, et al.: Treatment of childhood rhabdomyosarcoma at St. Jude Children's Research Hospital, 1962—1978. Natl Cancer Inst Monogr 56:93—101, 1981.
21. Ghavimi F, Exelby PR, D'Angio GJ, et al.: Multidisciplinary treatment of embryonal rhabdomyosarcoma in children. Cancer 35:677—686, 1975.
22. Maurer HM, Gehan EA, Beltangady M, et al.: The Intergroup Rhabdomyosarcoma Study II. Cancer, in press.
23. Maurer H, Gehan E, Crist W, et al.: Intergroup rhabdomyosarcoma study (IRS) III: A preliminary report of overall outcome. Proc Amer Soc Clin Oncol 8:296, 1989.
24. Kun L, Etcubanas E, Pratt C, et al.: Treatment factors affecting local control in childhood rhabdomyosarcoma (Abstr). Proc Am Soc Clin Oncol 5:207, 1986.
25. Tefft M, Wharam M, Gehan E: Local and regional control by radiation in IRS II. Int J Rad Oncol Biol Phys 16 (Suppl 1):159, 1988.
26. Crist WM, Raney RB, Ragab A, et al.: Intensive chemotherapy including cisplatin with and

without etoposide for children with soft tissue sarcomas. Med Pediatr Oncol 15:51—57, 1987.

27. Rao BN, Etcubanas EE, Horowitz M, et al.: The results of conservative management of extremity soft tissue sarcomas in children. Proc Ann Meet Am Soc Clin Oncol 5:266, 1986.

28. Brizel DM, Weinstein H, Hunt M, et al.: Failure pattern and survival in childhood soft tissue sarcomas. Proc Amer Soc Therapeut Radiat Oncol 29:183, 1988.

29. Mandell LR, Ghavini F, Exelby P, Fuks Z: Preliminary results of alternating combination chemotherapy (CT) and hyperfractionated radiotherapy (HART) in advanced rhabdomyosarcoma (RMS). Int J Radiat Oncol Biol Phys 15:197—203, 1988.

30. Carli M, Perilongo GT, Paolucci P, et al.: Role of primary chemotherapy in childhood malignant mesenchymal tumors other than rhabdomyosarcoma. Preliminary results. Proc Am Soc Clin Oncol 5:208, 1986.

31. Olive D, Famant F, Rodary C, et al.: Responsiveness of nonrhabdomyosarcoma malignant mesenchymal tumors (NRMMT) to primary chemotherapy (CT). Proc XXth Meeting SIOP, Trondheim, Norway, p 118, 1988.

32. Rosenberg SA, Tepper J, Glatstein E, et al.: Prospective randomized evaluation of adjuvant chemotherapy in adults with soft tissue sarcomas of the extremities. Cancer 52:424—434, 1983.

33. Antman K, Suit H, Amato D, et al.: Preliminary results of a randomized trial of adjuvant doxorubicin for sarcomas: Lack of apparent difference between treatment groups. J Clin Oncol 2:601—608, 1984.

34. Suit HD, Manken HJ, Schiller AL, et al.: Results of treatment of sarcomas of soft tissue by radiation and surgery at Massachusetts General Hospital. Cancer Treat Symp 3:43—47, 1985.

35. Bramwell VH, Mouridsen HT, Santoro A, et al.: Cyclophosphamide versus ifosfamide: Final report of a randomized Phase II trial in adult soft tissue sarcomas. Eur J Cancer Clin Oncol 23:311, 1987.

36. Stuart–Harris R, Harper PG, Kaye SB, Willshaw E: High-dose ifosfamide by infusion with mesna in advanced soft tissue sarcoma. Cancer Treat Rev 10 (Suppl A):163—164, 1983.

37. Suit HD: Patterns of failure after treatment of sarcoma of soft tissue by radical surgery or by conservative surgery and radiation. Cancer Treat Symp 2:241—246, 1983.

38. Potter DA, Glenn J, Kinsella T, et al.: Patterns of recurrence in patients with high-grade soft-tissue sarcomas. J Clin Oncol 3:353—366, 1985.

39. Collin C, Godbold J, Hajdu S, Brennan M: Localized extremity soft tissue sarcoma: An analysis of factors affecting survival. J Clin Oncol 5:601—612, 1987.

40. Roth JA, Putnam JB, Jr, Wesley MN, Rosenberg SA: Differing determinants of prognosis following resection of pulmonary metastasis from osteogenic and soft tissue sarcomas. Cancer 55:1361—1366, 1988.

41. Ueda T, Aozasa K, Tsujimoto M, et al.: Multivariate analysis for clinical prognostic factors in 163 patients with soft tissue sarcoma. Cancer 62:1444—1450, 1988.

42. Mandard AM, Petiot JF, Marnay J, et al.: Prognostic factors in soft tissue sarcomas: A multivariate analysis of 109 cases. Cancer 63:1437—1451, 1989.

43. Shiraki M, Enterline HT, Brooks JJ, et al.: Pathologic analysis of advanced adult soft tissue sarcomas, bone sarcomas and mesotheliomas. The Eastern Cooperative Oncology Group (ECOG) experience. Cancer 64:484—490, 1989.

44. Eilber FR, Morton DL, Eckardt J, et al.: Limb salvage for skeletal and soft tissue sarcomas: Multidisciplinary preoperative therapy. Cancer 53:2579—2584, 1984.

45. Lindberg RD, Martin RG, Romsdahl MM, Barkley HT, Jr: Conservative surgery and postoperative radiotherapy in 300 adults with soft tissue sarcomas. Cancer 47:2391—2397, 1981.

46. Slater JD, McNeese MD, Peters LJ: Radiation therapy for unresectable soft tissue sarcomas. Int J Radiat Oncol Biol Phys 12:1729—1734, 1986.

47. Suit HD, Maukin HJ, Wood WC, Proppe KH: Preoperative, intraoperative, and postoperative radiation in the treatment of primary soft tissue sarcoma. Cancer 55:2659—2667, 1985.

163

48. Fontanesi J, Kun L, Pao W, et al.: Brachytherapy as primary or "boost" irradiation in 18 children with solid tumors. Int J Endocurie Therapy/Hyperthermia Oncol, submitted.
49. Curran WJ, Jr, Littman P, Raney RB: Interstitial radiation therapy in the treatment of childhood soft-tissue sarcomas. Int J Radiat Oncol Biol Phys 14:169—174, 1988.
50. Knight PJ, Doornbos JF, Rosen D, et al.: The use of interstitial radiation therapy in the treatment of persistent, localized, and unresectable cancer in children. Cancer 57:951—954, 1986.
51. Pratt C, James DH, Holton CP, Pinkel D: Combination therapy including vincristine for malignant solid tumors in children. Cancer Chemother Rep 52:489—495, 1968.
52. Pinkel D: Cyclophosphamide in children with cancer. Cancer 15:42—49, 1962.
53. Pinkel D: Actinomycin D in childhood cancer: A preliminary report. Pediatrics 23:342—347, 1959.
54. Gottlieb JA, Baker LH, O'Bryan RM, et al.: Adriamycin (NSC-123127) used alone and in combination for soft tissue and bony sarcomas. Cancer Chemother Rep 6 (Pt 3):271—282, 1975.
55. Tan C, Rosen G, Ghavimi F, et al.: Adriamycin (NSC-123127) in pediatric malignancies. Cancer Chemother Rep 6 (Pt 3):259—266, 1975.
56. Gottlieb JA, Benjamin RS, Baker LM, et al.: Role of DTIC (NSC-45388) in the chemotherapy of sarcomas. Cancer Treat Rep 60:199—203, 1976.
57. Pratt CB, Hayes FA, Green AA, et al.: Pharmacokinetic evaluation of cisplatin in children with malignant solid tumors. A phase II study. Cancer Treat Rep 65:1021—1026, 1981.
58. O'Dwyer PJ, Leyland–Jones B, Alonso MT, et al.: Etoposide (VP-16,213): Current status of an active anticancer drug. N Engl J Med 312:692—700, 1985.
59. Magrath I, Sandlund J, Raynor A, et al.: A phase II study of ifosfamide in the treatment of recurrent sarcomas in young people. Cancer Chemother Pharmacol 18 (Suppl 2):S25—S28, 1985.
60. Pratt CB, Douglass EC, Goren MP, et al.: Clinical studies of ifosfamide/mesna at St. Jude Children's Research Hospital, 1983—1988. Semin Oncol 16 (Suppl 3):51—55, 1989.
61. Grier HE, Perez–Atayde AR, Weinstein HJ: Chemotherapy for inoperable infantile fibrosarcoma. Cancer 56:1507—1510, 1985.
62. Horowitz M, Balis F, Pastakia B, et al.: Integration of ifosfamide and VP-16 (IE) into the frontline therapy of pediatric sarcomas (PS). Proc Ann Meet Am Soc Clin Oncol 7:260, 1988.
63. Castello MA, Clerico A, Jenkner A, Dominici C: High-dose carboplatin and etoposide in children with malignant solid tumors. Proc XXth Meeting SIOP, Trondheim, Norway, p 195, 1988.
64. Miser JS, Kinsella TJ, Triche TJ, et al.: Ifosfamide with Mesna uroprotection and etoposide: An effective regimen in the treatment of recurrent sarcomas and other tumors of children and young adults. J Clin Oncol 5:1191—1198, 1987.
65. Edmonson JH, Fleming TR, Ivins JC, et al.: Randomized study of systemic chemotherapy following complete excision of non-osseous sarcoma. J Clin Oncol 2:1390—1396, 1984.
66. de Paula U, Suit HD, Harmon D: Adjuvant chemotherapy in clinical stage M_0 sarcoma of soft tissue. Cancer 62:1907—1911, 1988.
67. Flamant F, Rodary C, Rey A, Praquin MT: Preliminary report on the SIOP protocol for malignant mesenchymal tumors. Proc XVIIth Meeting SIOP, Venice, Italy, pp 81—84, 1985.
68. Kung FH, Pratt CD, Krischer JP: Ifosfamide and VP-16 in the treatment of recurrent malignant solid tumors of childhood. Proc Ann Meet Am Soc Clin Oncol 8:301, 1989.
69. Stout AP: Fibrosarcoma in infants and children. Cancer 5:1028—1040, 1962.
70. Soule EH, Pritchard DJ: Fibrosarcoma of infants and children: A review of 110 cases. Cancer 40:1711—1721, 1977.
71. Ninane J, Gosseye S, Panteon E, et al.: Congenital fibrosarcoma: Preoperative chemotherapy and conservative surgery. Cancer 58:1400—1406, 1986.

164

72. Blocker S, Koenig J, Ternberg J: Congenital fibrosarcoma. J. Pediatr Surg 22:665—670, 1987.
73. Gansar GF, Krementz ET: Desmoid tumors: Experience with new modes of therapy. South Med J 81:794—796, 1988.
74. Raney RB: Synovial sarcoma. Med Pediatr Oncol 9:41—45, 1981.
75. Kauffman SL, Stout AP: Hemangiopericytoma in children. Cancer 13:695—710, 1960.
76. Shmookler BM, Enzinger FM: Juvenile liposarcoma: An analysis of 15 cases. Am J Clin Pathol 133:245—246, 1982.
77. Weiss SW, Enzinger FM: Malignant fibrous histiocytoma: An analysis of 200 cases. Cancer 41:2250—2266, 1978.
78. Raney RB, Allen A, O'Neill J, et al.: Malignant fibrous histiocytoma of soft tissue in childhood. Cancer 57:2198—2201, 1986.
79. Mayer CMH, Favara BE, Holton CP, Rainer G: Malignant mesenchymoma in infants. Am J Dis Child 128:847—850, 1974.
80. Ducatman BS, Scheithauer BW, Piepgras DG, et al.: Malignant peripheral nerve sheath tumors: A clinicopathologic study of 120 cases. Cancer 57:2006—2021, 1986.
81. Raney RB, Schnaufer L, Zeigler M, et al.: Treatment of children with neurogenic sarcoma. Cancer 59:1—5, 1987.
82. Enzinger FM, Weiss SW: Malignant tumors of uncertain histogenesis. In: Soft tissue tumors, 2nd edition. Enzinger FM, Weiss SW, (eds). St Louis: CV Mosby, pp 929—965, 1988.
83. Nakashima Y, Unni KK, Shives TC, et al.: Mesenchymal chondrosarcoma of bone and soft tissue: A review of 111 cases. Cancer 57:2444—2453, 1986.
84. Chase DR, Enzinger FM: Epithelioid sarcoma: Diagnosis, prognostic indications and treatment. Am J Surg Pathd 9:241—263, 1985.
85. Kawamoto EH, Weidner N, Agostini RM, Jr, Jaffe R: Malignant ectomesenchymoma of soft tissue: Report of 2 cases and review of the literature. Cancer 59:1791—1802, 1987.
86. Soule EH, Newton W, Moon TE, Tefft M: Extraskeletal Ewing's sarcoma. Cancer 42:259—264, 1968.
87. Askin FB, Rosai J, Sibley RK, et al.: Malignant small cell tumor of the thoracopulmonary region in childhood: A distinctive clinicopathologic entity of uncertain histogenesis. Cancer 43:2438—2451, 1979.
88. Llombart–Bosch A, Lacombe MJ, Contesso G, Peydro–Olaya A: Small round blue cell sarcoma of bone mimicking atypical Ewing's sarcoma with neuroectodermal features. Cancer 60:1570—1582, 1987.
89. Shimada H, Newton W, Soule E, et al.: Pathologic features of extraosseous Ewing's sarcoma. Hum Pathol 19:422—453, 1988.
90. Cavazzana AD, Ninfo V, Montesco M, et al.: Peripheral neuroepithelioma: Morphologic and immunologic criteria for diagnosis (Abstr). Mod Pathol 1:17, 1988.
91. Marina NM, Etcubanas E, Parham D, et al.: Peripheral primitive neuroectodermal tumor (peripheral neuroepithelioma) in children: A review of the St. Jude experience and controversies in diagnosis and management. Cancer 64:1952—1960, 1989.
92. Laskin WB, Silverman TA, Enzinger FM: Postradiation soft tissue sarcomas: An analysis of 53 cases. Cancer 62:2330—2340, 1988.

Index

Ifosfamide (IFOS), 77–78, 79, 82–83, 85,
    86, 101
  hyperthermia and, 140
  for pediatric sarcomas, 158, 159
IL-2 (Interleukin-2), 79, 130
Imidazole carboxamide, see Decarbazine
Immunotherapy, 117
Incidence of sarcoma, 37, 105
  pediatric, 151–154
Incisional biopsies, 1, 41, 43, 154
Interferons, 79, 130, 141
Interleukin-2 (IL-2), 79, 130
Intimal dissections, 106
Intra-arterial chemotherapy, 65, 67, 85–86,
    105–111, 119, 134
Intracapsular resection, 157
Intralesional procedures, 44–45, 46
Intraoperative electron radiation therapy,
    69–70

Kaposi's sarcoma, 2, 3, 31
Karnofsky Performance Scale, 56

Large cell lymphomas, 3
Leiomyosarcomas, 2, 4, 5
  chemotherapy for, 84
  pediatric, 152, 153
  staging of, 32
  surgery for, 39
LET radiations, 70–71
Leukemia, 58
Leukocytopenia, 82
LH (Luteinizing hormone), 100
Lidocaine, 130
Limb-salvage procedures, 49, 99
  biopsies in, 41
  chemotherapy and, 105, 107, 109, 110,
    119
  diagnostic imaging and, 11
  psychological outcome of, 53–59
  radiation therapy and, 67
Lipoblasts, 2
Lipomas
  biopsies of, 43
  diagnostic imaging of, 16, 17, 18, 19, 23
  pleomorphic, 2
  surgery for, 37, 46, 50
Liposarcomas, 5
  biopsies of, 41
  chemotherapy for, 84, 114
  dedifferentiated, 5
  myxoid, 2, 3

  pediatric, 152, 153
  staging of, 32
  surgery for, 38, 39
Lobular hemangiomas, 3
Lonidamine, 128
Luteinizing hormone (LH), 100
Lymphangiograms, 40
Lymphatic sarcomas, 2, 114
Lymph node metastases
  chemotherapy for, 114
  of pediatric sarcomas, 149, 150, 154
  staging of, 33, 34
  surgery for, 39, 49
Lymphomas, 1, 3, 40, 58
Lymphoreticular cells, 4
Lysosomes, 127

Magnetic induction hyperthermia, 140
Magnetic resonance imaging (MRI), 12,
    14–16, 18–23, 24, 25, 26, 27
  surgery and, 40, 49
Malignant fibrous histiocytomas (MFH), 2,
    3, 4, 7
  chemotherapy for, 84, 111, 114
  diagnostic imaging of, 18, 20, 21, 25, 26
  pediatric, 152, 153, 160
  pleomorphic, 5
  staging of, 32
  surgery for, 38
Malignant lesions, see also specific types
  biopsies of, 43
  diagnostic imaging of, 23
  staging of, 34
  surgery for, 37, 38, 45, 46, 50
Malignant Mesenchymal Tumor (MMT)
    Protocol, 159
Marginal surgical procedures, 44, 45, 46, 47,
    95, 109, 157
Margins, 44–46
  radiation therapy and, 64–65, 72
MDMS, 78
MDR (Multidrug-resistant) phenotype, 76
Melanomas, 2, 3, 111
Melphalan, 115, 118, 119, 122, 130, 131, 133
Menogaril, 77
Menstruation, 100
Mesenchymal cells, 5, 31
Mesenchymal tumors, 1, 3, 32, 53
Mesna, 101, 159
Mesoderm, 149
Mesodermal sarcomas, 114
Mesotheliomas, 152, 153
Metastases